Phototherapy and Photodiagnostic Methods for the Practitioner

Phototherapy and Photodiagnostic Methods for the Practitioner

Editors

Wei-Sheng Chong
Jiun-Yit Pan
Eugene Sern-Ting Tan

National Skin Centre, Singapore

World Scientific

NEW JERSEY • LONDON • SINGAPORE • BEIJING • SHANGHAI • HONG KONG • TAIPEI • CHENNAI • TOKYO

Published by

World Scientific Publishing Co. Pte. Ltd.
5 Toh Tuck Link, Singapore 596224
USA office: 27 Warren Street, Suite 401-402, Hackensack, NJ 07601
UK office: 57 Shelton Street, Covent Garden, London WC2H 9HE

Library of Congress Cataloging-in-Publication Data
Names: Chong, Wei Sheng, editor. | Pan, Jiun Yit, editor. | Tan, Eugene Sern Ting, editor.
Title: Phototherapy and photodiagnostic methods for the practitioner / edited by
Wei Sheng Chong, Jiun Yit Pan & Sern Ting Eugene Tan.
Description: New Jersey : World Scientific, 2016. | Includes bibliographical references and index.
Identifiers: LCCN 2016029475 | ISBN 9789813146631 (hardcover : alk. paper)
Subjects: | MESH: Phototherapy | Photochemotherapy | Photosensitivity Disorders
Classification: LCC RM838 | NLM WB 480 | DDC 615.8/31--dc23
LC record available at https://lccn.loc.gov/2016029475

British Library Cataloguing-in-Publication Data
A catalogue record for this book is available from the British Library.

Typeset by Stallion Press
Email: enquiries@stallionpress.com

Printed in Singapore

Contents

Annexes

Editors

CHONG Wei Sheng
MBBS (Singapore), MMed (Int Med), MRCP (UK), FAMS (Dermatology), FRCP (Edinburgh)
Senior Consultant Dermatologist
National Skin Centre, Singapore
Dermatology Service, Khoo Teck Puat Hospital, Singapore

PAN Jiun Yit
MBBS (Singapore), MRCP (UK), DPD (Cardiff), Dip Derm (RCPSG), MCI (NUS), GDOM (NUS), DTM & H (London), FAMS (Dermatology), FRCP (Edinburgh)
Consultant Dermatologist
National Skin Centre, Singapore

TAN Sern Ting Eugene
MBBS (Singapore), DPD (Cardiff), Dip Derm (RCPSG), FAMS (Dermatology)
Consultant Dermatologist
National Skin Centre, Singapore

Contributors

CHONG Wei Sheng
MBBS (Singapore), MMed (Int Med), MRCP (UK), FAMS (Dermatology), FRCP (Edinburgh)
Senior Consultant Dermatologist
National Skin Centre, Singapore
Dermatology Service, Khoo Teck Puat Hospital, Singapore

HENG Yee Kiat
MBBS (Singapore), MMed (Int Med), MRCP (UK)
Consultant Dermatologist
National Skin Centre, Singapore

HO Ju Ee Sue-Ann
MBBS (Singapore), MRCP (UK), FAMS (Dermatology)
Consultant Dermatologist
Division of Dermatology, University Medicine Cluster
National University Health System, Singapore

LIM Kar Seng
MBBS (Singapore), MRCP (UK), FAMS (Dermatology)
Consultant Dermatologist
The Dermatology Practice, Singapore

OON Hwee Boon Hazel
MD (Toronto), MMed (Int Med), MRCP (UK), GDFM, FAMS (Dermatology)
Consultant Dermatologist
National Skin Centre, Singapore

PAN Jiun Yit
MBBS (Singapore), MRCP (UK), DPD (Cardiff), Dip Derm (RCPSG), MCI (NUS), GDOM (NUS), DTM & H (London), FAMS (Dermatology), FRCP (Edinburgh)
Consultant Dermatologist
National Skin Centre, Singapore

TAN Ki Wei
MBBS (Singapore), MRCP (UK)
Consultant Dermatologist
Department of Dermatology
Changi General Hospital, Singapore

TAN Sern Ting Eugene
MBBS (Singapore), DPD (Cardiff), Dip Derm (RCPSG), FAMS (Dermatology)
Consultant Dermatologist
National Skin Centre, Singapore

TAN Yoke Choo
SRN (Singapore)
Nurse Clinician
National Skin Centre, Singapore

THENG Thiam Seng Colin
MBBS (Singapore), MMed (Fam Med), MRCP (UK), FAMS (Dermatology)
Consultant Dermatologist
The Skin Specialists and Laser Clinic, Singapore

Foreword

by
Henry W. Lim, MD
C.S. Livingood Chair and Chairman
Department of Dermatology
Henry Ford Hospital
Detroit, Michigan, US

Photodermatology is an integral and essential part of dermatology. It is a discipline that is a part of the curriculum of a dermatology training programme, and it is used in our clinical practice daily. This book is a timely one as it focuses on practical treatment protocols for phototherapy and for the diagnosis of photodermatoses in Asian skin. The editors are to be congratulated in organising the book in an easy-to-read and practical format.

While there are several textbooks on photodermatology, a widely referenced treatment protocol textbook was published in the United States in 2000. Asia is a rapidly growing demographic group worldwide. The distribution of photodermatoses in Asia, especially in countries closer to the equator, is different from that seen in countries with temperate climates with a predominantly fair-skinned population.

The National Skin Centre (NSC) in Singapore is a widely recognised centre of excellence in dermatology. It serves as a referral centre for the region, and attracts trainees worldwide. The editors and the authors have drawn on their collective clinical experience at NSC to prepare this book. It would serve as a practical reference for all dermatologists, trainees, nurses and other professionals in the delivery of high-quality phototherapy, and for dermatologists and trainees in the evaluation of patients with photodermatoses.

Foreword

by
Robert P.E. Sarkany, BSc (Hons), MBBS (Hons), FRCP, MD
Head of Photodermatology Unit
St John's Institute of Dermatology
London, UK

Photodermatology has gone through a revolution in recent decades, with a transformation of the understanding of the effects of ultraviolet light on the skin. Yet, for the clinician, photodermatology remains a practical subspecialty. Effective phototherapy and accurate photodiagnosis depend on clinical staff using reliable, precise and correct methodology.

Phototherapy and Photodiagnostic Methods for the Practitioner is a welcome practical reference to guide dermatologists and others working in clinical photodermatology. Many clinicians are put off by this fascinating and clinically important area because they feel ill-equipped to tackle the complexities of ultraviolet light sources and dosage protocols. This book gives clear evidence-based answers to the questions a clinician will face in the clinic when managing patients in phototherapy and photodiagnosis, and provides a straightforward practical manual to enable clinicians to set up and do the key phototherapeutic and photodiagnostic procedures. It is also a delight to see this book finally filling the long-standing deficiency in the literature as the first published set of practical guidelines for patients with Asian skin.

This book will sit on the bookshelf in my clinic for the clinical team to consult. If you are just starting out on the endlessly fascinating path of clinical photodermatology, this book will clear the fog that can sometimes obscure the way.

Preface

by
CHONG Wei Sheng, FRCP
PAN Jiun Yit, FRCP
TAN Sern Ting Eugene, FAMS

Phototherapy is an important modality in a dermatologist's therapeutic armamentarium, with established efficacy for a number of common skin diseases such as atopic dermatitis, psoriasis and vitiligo. The accurate diagnosis of a photodermatosis relies on a good clinical history and physical examination, supported by photodiagnostic investigations such as phototesting as appropriate.

To our knowledge, *Phototherapy and Photodiagnostic Methods for the Practitioner* is the first published set of practical guidelines pertaining to the use of phototherapy and photodiagnostic testing in Asian skin. The book draws upon our cumulative clinical experience with phototherapy for various dermatoses at the National Skin Centre in Singapore over the years, amalgamated with up-to-date evidence from the scientific literature. It is designed to serve as a concise and comprehensive reference manual for dermatologists in Asia, as well as other clinicians and nurses with an interest in photodiagnostic investigations and phototherapy for the evaluation and treatment of skin disorders.

We would like to thank our contributors for their valuable input in the various chapters, and trust you will find this book a useful and enjoyable read.

Chapter

1

Introduction to Phototherapy

- Phototherapy and photochemotherapy are established modalities of treatment for a variety of skin diseases, including atopic dermatitis, psoriasis, vitiligo and mycosis fungoides.
- The therapeutic effect is based on the interaction between ultraviolet radiation (UVR) and the skin, and is believed to be via the induction of immunosuppression and T-cell apoptosis, leading to cell-cycle arrest in hyperproliferating cells such as the keratinocytes.
- Phototherapy is the therapeutic use of UVR without the use of an exogenous photosensitiser.

- Photochemotherapy (psoralen with ultraviolet A or PUVA) involves the combined use of the drug psoralen with ultraviolet A (UVA) radiation. Psoralen, given topically or orally, acts as a photosensitiser to enhance the effect of UVA.

Chapter

2

Nursing Considerations in Phototherapy

Pre-Phototherapy Advice

- The patient should be advised that multiple sessions of phototherapy would be required before clinical improvement is seen. For instance, an average of 20 to 25 sessions of narrowband ultraviolet B (NBUVB) phototherapy is required for effective treatment of psoriasis. Regular irradiation of up to three times a week is required, especially in the initial clearing phase of treatment. The patient should also be advised that irregular treatments may affect and delay a successful outcome.
- The first exposure is usually short, lasting seconds to a minute, depending on the person's Fitzpatrick skin phototype.

- The objective is to apply the largest phototherapy dose that causes mild, asymptomatic erythema. Once this is reached, further doses will be adjusted to maintain this mild, asymptomatic erythema.
- Once the patient is lesion-free, the maintenance phase with reduction in frequency of treatment will commence.
- Applying an emollient such as liquid paraffin on the skin before irradiation increases UVR permeability and hence the therapeutic effect, especially in the context of psoriasis treatment. However, the use of extremely greasy and opaque ointments may impede UVR permeability.

NBUVB Treatment Procedure

Pre-NBUVB Irradiation

1. Explain the treatment procedure and side effects of NBUVB phototherapy, and obtain informed consent.
2. A shower prior to NBUVB phototherapy can aid in reducing skin scaling, especially in psoriasis.
3. Prior to irradiation, assess the skin condition for
   a. Extent and severity of involvement.
   b. Response of lesional and non-lesional skin to previous treatment.

During NBUVB Irradiation

1. A thin layer of liquid paraffin is applied to the scaly lesions to help in enhancing NBUVB penetration and its therapeutic effect.
2. Ensure that the male patient wears protective gear to cover the genital area.
3. The patient and nurse must wear UV-protective goggles.

4. Protect the patient's face with a covering hood, unless the face requires irradiation. For patients with long hair, tie the hair above the neck at all times during each treatment session.

5. An additional hand-held safety timer will be set for each treatment session, corresponding to the time calculated for the NBUVB dose for that treatment.

Post-NBUVB Treatment Advice

1. Warn the patient that erythema and mild skin discomfort may appear after treatment. Such effects are easily relieved by a cold shower and the application of a cold moisturiser. However, if more severe reactions such as pain, swelling and blistering develop, the patient should be advised to consult the doctor immediately.

2. Minimise further exposure to natural UVR from the sun by wearing a long-sleeved shirt with long pants or carrying an umbrella when going outdoors, and by applying a sunscreen.

3. Continue the usual topical treatment as prescribed.

4. Record the dose and the time of NBUVB delivered, and the progress of the patient's condition.

Oral PUVA Treatment Procedure

Pre-UVA Irradiation

1. Explain the treatment procedure and side effects of PUVA photochemotherapy, and obtain informed consent.

2. A shower prior to PUVA photochemotherapy can aid in reducing skin scaling, especially in psoriasis.

3. Ensure that the patient has taken the prescribed dose of 8-methoxypsoralen (8-MOP) tablets (Meladinine®, CLS Pharma) two hours before the scheduled treatment time. This serves to

increase the sensitivity of the skin to UVA radiation. The effect of the medication peaks approximately two hours after oral ingestion.

4. Prior to irradiation, assess the skin condition for
   a. Extent and severity of involvement.
   b. Response of lesional and non-lesional skin to previous treatment.

During UVA Irradiation

1. A thin layer of liquid paraffin is applied to the scaly lesions to help in enhancing UVA penetration and its therapeutic effect.
2. Ensure that the male patient wears protective gear to cover the genital area.
3. The patient and nurse must wear UV-protective goggles.
4. Protect the patient's face with a covering hood, unless the face requires irradiation. For patients with long hair, tie the hair above the neck at all times during each treatment session.
5. An additional hand-held safety timer will be set for each treatment session, corresponding to the time calculated for the UVA dose for that treatment.

Post-PUVA Treatment Advice

1. Warn the patient that erythema and mild skin discomfort may appear after treatment. Such effects are easily relieved by a cold shower and the application of a cold moisturiser. However, if more severe reactions such as pain, swelling and blistering develop, the patient should be advised to consult the doctor immediately.
2. Minimise further exposure to natural UVR from the sun by wearing UV-protective sunglasses (must be worn for 24 hours after ingestion of oral 8-MOP) and a long-sleeved shirt with long pants, or carrying an umbrella when going outdoors, and by applying a sunscreen.
3. Continue the usual topical treatment as prescribed.

4. Record the dose and the time of UVA delivered, and the progress of the patient's condition.

Bath/Soak/Paint PUVA Treatment Procedure

There are a few differences between bath/soak/paint and oral PUVA photochemotherapies:

- Instead of ingesting 8-MOP tablets, in bath PUVA photochemotherapy, the patient is bathed in warm water with 8-MOP solution added to a final concentration of 3.75 mg/L at 37°C.
- In soak PUVA photochemotherapy, the patient's hands and/or feet are soaked in water with 8-MOP solution added to a final concentration of 3.75 mg/L.
- In paint PUVA photochemotherapy, 8-MOP solution is applied as a thin layer with a cotton swab to lesional skin, taking care to avoid applying to surrounding unaffected skin.
- In bath and soak PUVA photochemotherapies, the patient is soaked for 20 minutes. Keep the water circulating to maintain homogeneous concentration of the diluted 8-MOP. Subsequently, the patient is exposed to UVA radiation immediately, or within 15 minutes.
- In paint PUVA photochemotherapy, after applying the 8-MOP solution to the lesional skin, wait for a further 20 minutes before UVA irradiation.
- After UVA irradiation, the patient must thoroughly wash off any remaining 8-MOP that is left on the skin.
- There is no need to wear UV-protective sunglasses after completing bath/soak/paint PUVA photochemotherapies. However, the patient should minimise further exposure to natural UVR from the sun by wearing a long-sleeved shirt with long pants, or carrying an umbrella when going outdoors, and by applying a sunscreen.

Chapter

3

Narrowband Ultraviolet B Phototherapy

Background

- Narrowband ultraviolet B (NBUVB) refers to a specific spectrum of UVR with a wavelength of 311 ± 2 nm. After Fischer's initial discovery that UVR of wavelength 313 nm achieved clearance of psoriatic plaques, further studies showed that UVB was most therapeutically effective at 311 nm, superior to broadband UVB (BBUVB).
- NBUVB acts mainly in the epidermis and basal layer, and exerts a number of local immunosuppressive effects.
- Over the years, NBUVB has established itself as a relatively safe and cost-effective therapeutic modality and is widely used for the treatment of extensive psoriasis and other UVB-responsive dermatoses (Figure 1).

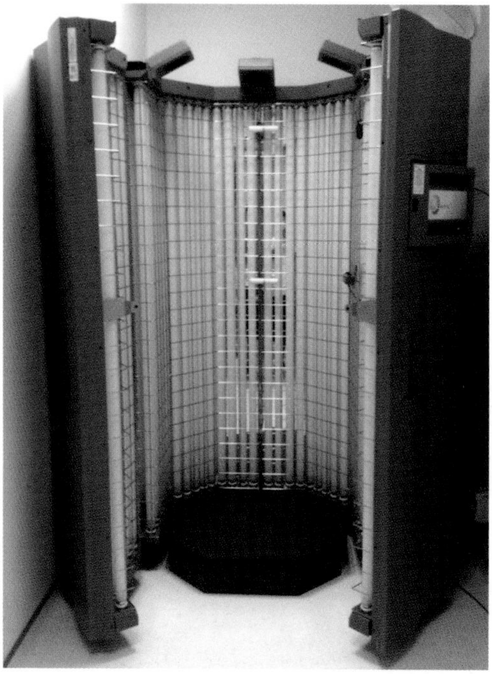

Figure 1. Narrowband UVB phototherapy cabin.

Indications of NBUVB Phototherapy

General

- Extensive skin lesions on trunk and limbs rendering topical therapy impractical
- Failure of topical therapy

Common

• Psoriasis	[A, Ib]
• Atopic dermatitis	[A, Ib]
• Vitiligo	[A, Ib]
• Mycosis fungoides	[B, IIa]

Others [C, IV]

- Nodular prurigo
- Pityriasis rosea
- Pityriasis lichenoides chronica

- Generalised pruritus (e.g. in renal failure)
- Lichen planus
- Chronic spontaneous urticaria
- Progressive macular hypomelanosis

Contraindications to NBUVB Phototherapy

Absolute

- Severe medical illness that prevents standing in the phototherapy cabin
- Haemodynamic instability
- Systemic lupus erythematosus, dermatomyositis
- Genophotodermatoses (e.g. xeroderma pigmentosum)
- Photosensitivity
- Personal history of melanoma

Relative

- Personal history of non melanoma skin cancer (NMSC)
- Pre-malignant skin lesions (e.g. actinic keratosis)
- Atypical naevus syndrome
- Family history of skin cancer
- Previous exposure to arsenic or ionising radiation
- Poorly controlled epilepsy
- Photosensitising drugs
- Treatment with immunosuppressive drugs that significantly increase the risk of skin cancer (e.g. ciclosporin)

Adverse Effects of NBUVB Phototherapy

Acute

- Pruritus
- Erythema
- Blistering
- Pigmentation (Tanning)
- Aggravation of existing skin disease
- Provocation of polymorphic light eruption (PMLE)

Chronic

- Premature photoageing
- Skin malignancy, especially squamous cell carcinoma (SCC)

Treatment Regimen and Dosimetry

Treatment Initiation

- NBUVB phototherapy is started at a frequency of two to three times per week.
- The objective is to deliver a suberythemogenic dose of NBUVB to achieve the best therapeutic response. The initial NBUVB dose (mJ/cm^2) can be determined by one of two approaches:

Approach #1: MED Regimen [A, Ib]

- The patient's minimal erythema dose (MED) is determined prior to commencing NBUVB phototherapy. The MED regimen is individually tailored and considered to be the safest and most optimal dosimetry for the patient.
- We routinely use 70% of MED as the initial NBUVB dose. Refer to Chapter 9 — Phototesting and Annex A for details of MED testing and the dosimetry respectively.

Initial NBUVB dose = 70% of MED

Approach #2: Skin Phototype Regimen [C, IV]

- This method, based on skin phototype, is generally used in a patient whose skin disease is so extensive that there is inadequate normal skin for MED testing.
- In practice, this method is more convenient and preferred in some busy phototherapy centres with a heavy patient load, as it may be impractical to conduct MED testing for every patient.

- The definitions of the various Fitzpatrick skin phototypes and the starting dosimetry used are summarised in the following two tables.

Skin Phototype	**Colour of Skin and Hair**	**Ethnic Descent**	**Sunburn**	**Tanning**
I	Very fair skin, freckles, red hair	Celtic type	Always	Never
II	Skin slightly darker, hair blond to brown	Fair-skinned European	Easily	Mild
III	Skin fair to light-brown, hair dark-blond, brown to black	Medium-brown European, fair-skinned Asian	Moderate	Moderate
IV	Skin light-brown to olive-coloured, hair dark-brown to black	Mediterranean European, Chinese, Malay, North-Indian	Minimal	Deep
V	Skin brown, hair dark-brown to black	Middle-East type, darker-skinned Asian, Indian	Rare	Rapid, deep
VI	Skin dark-brown, hair black	African, South-Indian	Never	Always dark

Skin Phototype	**Initial NBUVB Dose (mJ/cm^2)**
I	300
II	400
III	500
IV	600
V	700
VI	800

Dose Adjustment Based on Erythema [C, IV]

- The goal of phototherapy is to maintain a mild, just perceptible erythema throughout the treatment course.
- On each subsequent visit, the patient's severity of erythema is assessed in order to determine the dose adjustment (as shown in the following table). Depending on the erythema response, the dose of NBUVB is usually increased with each session to counteract the effects of photoadaptation due to the phototherapy, namely epidermal hyperplasia and pigmentation (tanning).

Erythema History	Erythema Grading	Description of Erythema on Attendance	Dose Adjustment
None	0	No erythema	↑by 20% of MED or 100 mJ/cm^2
< 48 hours	±	No erythema (erythema is reported only by patient)	↑by 10% of MED or 50 mJ/cm^2
48–72 hours	+	Just perceptible pink erythema, asymptomatic	Hold dose
≥ 48–72 hours	++	Well-defined erythema, possibly causing slight manageable discomfort	↓by 25% of previous dose, or postpone treatment. When settled, restart after three days at previous dose.
Painful without blistering	+++	Well-defined fiery-red erythema, symptomatic, painful	No treatment. Review by doctor. When settled, restart after one week at 50% of previous dose.
Painful with blistering	++++	Well-defined fiery-red, painful erythema with blistering	No treatment. Review by doctor. When settled, restart after one week at 50% of previous dose.

- If lesions on the lower legs and feet appear slow to respond, give them an additional 20% to 30% of the total body dose, with the rest of the body covered, and the patient standing on a platform of 12 to 16-cm height.

Maximum Dose per Session based on Skin Phototype [C, IV]

- The maximum NBUVB dose delivered per session should not be exceeded unless otherwise considered, as shown in the table below.

Skin Phototype	**Maximum NBUVB Dose (mJ/cm^2)**
I	4000
II	4000
III	5000
IV	5000
V	6000
VI	6000

Missed Treatment Protocol [C, IV]

- If a patient's treatment is missed or cancelled, the NBUVB dose should be adjusted accordingly as shown in the table below, based on the treatment interval between the previous and current sessions. In a situation when treatment is omitted due to erythema, the dose adjustment protocol based on erythema should be followed instead.

Treatment Interval (days)	**Dose Adjustment**
1 to 7	Hold dose or ↑dose as per protocol
8 to 14	↓dose by 25% of previous dose
15 to 21	↓dose by 50% of previous dose
22 to 28	↓dose by 75% of previous dose
> 28	Refer back to doctor, start over

<u>Expected Outcomes</u> [C, IV]

- In most cases, there should be a significant response expected after multiple treatment sessions, for instance, after 20 to 25 sessions in the case of psoriasis. If response is poor despite compliance with therapy, add or consider other modalities of treatment. The following table can be used as a guide for counselling patients on the expected outcomes in NBUVB phototherapy.

Diagnosis	**Estimated Number of Treatments**
Psoriasis	20–25
Eczema	30–35
Mycosis fungoides	25–30
Vitiligo	150–200 (commencement of repigmentation after 15–20 sessions)

<u>Maintenance Therapy</u> [C, IV]

- After the skin lesions have cleared or markedly improved (e.g. > 75% improvement), the patient may be continued on maintenance therapy to prevent a relapse of the disease. If the patient has started NBUVB phototherapy three times per week during the clearing phase of treatment, depending on the response, the frequency of treatment sessions may be gradually reduced to two times per week for several weeks, followed by once per week for several weeks, and the treatment is then stopped finally.
- For some patients, the disease relapses soon after the treatment is terminated, or alternative treatment modalities are not available or contraindicated. In such cases, once per fortnight maintenance therapy may be continued for several weeks or even months to keep the skin disease under control.
- The following table shows a general guideline for NBUVB dosimetry in these situations.

Tapered Frequency of Treatment	Dose Adjustment
Once per week	Hold dose
Once every two weeks (up to 12 months)	↓dose by 25% of previous dose and hold

Retinoid-NBUVB (Re-NBUVB) Treatment Regimen and Dosimetry [C, IV]

- The combination of a systemic retinoid such as acitretin and NBUVB phototherapy is best done using the MED regimen. In Re-NBUVB phototherapy, the initiation of the retinoid therapy should be done prior to the commencement of NBUVB treatment. In this case, the retinoid is initiated for a period of two weeks before performing NBUVB phototesting to determine the MED-Re-NBUVB. Obtaining the MED at this time gives a more accurate and effective dose of NBUVB and prevents phototoxic reactions from the treatment.
- However, when phototesting to determine MED-Re-NBUVB is not feasible, skin phototype regimen is then used with the starting dose of NBUVB equivalent to 50% of the original initial NBUVB dose based on the respective skin phototype.
- In the case when the systemic retinoid is started after the patient has already undergone induction of NBUVB phototherapy, then the dose of NBUVB is maintained for a period of two weeks after the introduction of the retinoid, followed by subsequent dose adjustment based on the erythema response.

Skin Cancer Surveillance for Patients on Long-Term NBUVB Phototherapy [C, IV]

- As with other phototherapies, there is no clear-cut evidence on which to base a recommendation for a maximum lifetime number of treatments.

- Patients receiving more than 500 NBUVB treatment sessions should be considered as possibly being at increased risk of skin cancer and managed accordingly with regular skin cancer surveillance and close monitoring for skin malignancy.

Further Reading

1. Bandow GD, Koo JY. Narrow-band ultraviolet B radiation:A review of the current literature. *Int J Dermatol* 2004; 43: 555–561.
2. Cameron H, Dawe RS, Yule S, *et al.* A randomized, observer-blinded trial of twice vs. three times weekly narrowband ultraviolet B phototherapy for chronic plaque psoriasis. *Br J Dermatol* 2002; 147: 973–978.
3. Coven TR, Burack LH, Gilleaudeau R, *et al.* Narrowband UV-B produces superior clinical and histopathological resolution of moderate-to-severe psoriasis in patients compared with broadband UV-B. *Arch Dermatol* 1997; 133: 1514–1522.
4. Fischer T. Comparative treatment of psoriasis with UV-light, trioxsalen plus UV-light, and coal tar plus UV-light. *Acta Derm Venereol* 1977; 57: 345–350.
5. Gambichler T, Breuckmann F, Boms S, *et al.* Narrowband UVB phototherapy in skin conditions beyond psoriasis. *J Am Acad Dermatol* 2005; 52: 660–670.
6. Grundmann-Kollmann M, Behrens S, Podda M, *et al.* Phototherapy for atopic eczema with narrow-band UVB. *J Am Acad Dermatol* 1999; 40: 995–997.
7. Ibbotson SH, Bilsland D, Cox NH, *et al.* An update and guidance on narrowband ultraviolet B phototherapy: A British photodermatology group workshop report. *Br J Dermatol* 2004; 151: 283–297.
8. Kist JM, Van Voorhees AS. Narrowband ultraviolet B therapy for psoriasis and other skin disorders. *Adv Dermatol* 2005; 21: 235–250.
9. Scherschun L, Kim JJ, Lim HW. Narrow-band ultraviolet B is a useful and well-tolerated treatment for vitiligo. *J Am Acad Dermatol* 2001; 44: 999–1003.
10. Trautinger F. Phototherapy of mycosis fungoides. *Photodermatol Photoimmunol Photomed* 2011; 27: 68–74.
11. Zanolli MD, Feldman SR. *Phototherapy Treatment Protocols for Psoriasis and Other Phototherapy-Responsive Dermatoses*, 2nd ed. New York: Taylor & Francis Group; 2004.

Chapter

4

Combined Ultraviolet A/Narrowband Ultraviolet B Phototherapy

Background

- Combined ultraviolet A/narrowband ultraviolet B (UVA/NBUVB) phototherapy is another effective phototherapy modality that is useful for atopic dermatitis, apart from NBUVB itself.
- The earliest evidence for its efficacy can be traced back to the 1980s, when the currently antiquated broadband UVB (BBUVB) phototherapy machines were still being used. Back then, combined UVA/BBUVB phototherapy was shown to be more effective than BBUVB phototherapy alone for the treatment of severe atopic dermatitis. As NBUVB progressively superseded BBUVB

from the 1990s due to the former's superior efficacy and safety, combined UVA/NBUVB phototherapy was added to the photodermatologist's armamentarium.

- In our experience, the combined UVA/NBUVB phototherapy modality is found to be an effective and well-tolerated treatment option for pruritic dermatoses such as atopic dermatitis, nodular prurigo and chronic pruritus of various underlying aetiologies such as renal pruritus due to end-stage renal disease.
- The combined UVA/NBUVB phototherapy is particularly useful in patients who are intolerant to NBUVB phototherapy as the NBUVB dose used in the former is generally lower than that used in the latter.
- However, there is currently a paucity of quality evidence in the dermatology literature on the use of combined UVA/NBUVB phototherapy in pruritic dermatoses, particularly on how it compares with NBUVB in the treatment of atopic dermatitis. This may be due to the fact that combined UVA/NBUVB phototherapy modality is at present not widely available.
- Nevertheless, a small prospective observational study of 26 adult patients with chronic atopic dermatitis showed that the efficacy of UVA/NBUVB phototherapy was similar to that of NBUVB phototherapy.

Indications of Combined UVA/NBUVB Phototherapy

Main

- Atopic dermatitis [B, IIb]

Others [C, IV]

- Nodular prurigo
- Generalised pruritus (e.g. in renal failure)
- Aquagenic pruritus
- Pityriasis lichenoides

Contraindications to Combined UVA/NBUVB Phototherapy

Absolute

- Severe medical illness that prevents standing in the phototherapy cabin
- Haemodynamic instability
- Systemic lupus erythematosus, dermatomyositis
- Genophotodermatoses (e.g. xeroderma pigmentosum)
- Photosensitivity
- Personal history of melanoma

Relative

- Personal history of non-melanoma skin cancer (NMSC)
- Pre-malignant skin lesions (e.g. actinic keratosis)
- Atypical naevus syndrome
- Family history of skin cancer
- Previous exposure to arsenic or ionising radiation
- Poorly controlled epilepsy
- Photosensitising drugs
- Treatment with immunosuppressive drugs that significantly increase the risk of skin cancer (e.g. ciclosporin)

Adverse Effects of Combined UVA/NBUVB Phototherapy

Acute

- Pruritus
- Erythema
- Blistering
- Pigmentation (Tanning)
- Aggravation of existing skin disease
- Provocation of polymorphic light eruption (PMLE)

Chronic

- Premature photoageing
- Skin malignancy, especially squamous cell carcinoma (SCC)

Treatment Regimen and Dosimetry

Treatment Initiation

- Combined UVA/NBUVB phototherapy is started at a frequency of two to three times per week.

Dosimetry [C, IV]

- The dosimetry is based on the Fitzpatrick skin phototype. The following table shows the starting dosimetry.

Skin Phototype	Initial UVA Dose (J/cm^2)	Initial NBUVB Dose (mJ/cm^2)
I	1	50
II	2	100
III	3	150
IV	4	200
V	5	250
VI	6	300

Dose Adjustment Based on Erythema [C, IV]

- The goal of phototherapy is to maintain a mild, just perceptible erythema throughout the treatment course.
- On each subsequent visit, the patient's severity of erythema is assessed in order to determine the dose adjustment (as shown in the following table). Depending on the erythema response, the UVA and NBUVB doses are usually increased with each session to counteract the effects of photoadaptation due to the

phototherapy, namely epidermal hyperplasia and pigmentation (tanning).

Erythema History	Erythema Grading	Description of Erythema on Attendance	Dose Adjustment
None	0	No erythema	UVA: ↑ by 1 J/cm^2 NBUVB: ↑ by 100 mJ/cm^2
< 48 hours	±	No erythema (erythema is reported only by patient)	UVA: ↑ by 0.5 J/cm^2 NBUVB: ↑ by 50 mJ/cm^2
48–72 hours	+	Just perceptible pink erythema, asymptomatic	Hold dose
≥ 48–72 hours	++	Well-defined erythema, possibly causing slight manageable discomfort	↓ by 25% of previous dose, or postpone treatment. When settled, restart after three days at previous dose.
Painful without blistering	+++	Well-defined fiery-red erythema, symptomatic, painful	No treatment. Review by doctor. When settled, restart after one week at 50% of previous dose.
Painful with blistering	++++	Well-defined fiery-red, painful erythema with blistering	No treatment. Review by doctor. When settled, restart after one week at 50% of previous dose.

- If lesions on the lower legs and feet appear slow to respond, give them an additional 20% to 30% of the total body dose, with the rest of the body covered, and the patient standing on a platform of 12 to 16-cm height.

Maximum Dose per Session based on Skin Phototype [C, IV]

- The maximum UVA and NBUVB doses delivered per session should not be exceeded unless otherwise considered, as shown in the table below.

Skin Phototype	Maximum UVA Dose (J/cm^2)	Maximum NBUVB Dose (mJ/cm^2)
I	20	1000
II	20	1000
III	30	1500
IV	30	1500
V	40	2000
VI	40	2000

Missed Treatment Protocol [C, IV]

- If a patient's treatment is missed or cancelled, the UVA and NBUVB doses should be adjusted accordingly as shown in the table below, based on the treatment interval between the previous and current sessions. In a situation when treatment is omitted due to erythema, the dose adjustment protocol based on erythema should be followed instead.

Treatment Interval (days)	Dose Adjustment
1 to 7	Hold dose or ↑ dose as per protocol
8 to 14	↓ dose by 25% of previous dose
15 to 21	↓ dose by 50% of previous dose
22 to 28	↓ dose by 75% of previous dose
> 28	Refer back to doctor, start over

Maintenance Therapy [C, IV]

- After the skin lesions have cleared or markedly improved (e.g. >75% improvement), the patient may be continued on maintenance therapy to prevent a relapse of the disease. If the patient has started the combined UVA/NBUVB phototherapy three times per week during the clearing phase of treatment, depending on the response, the frequency of treatment sessions may be gradually reduced to two times per week for several weeks, followed by once per week for several weeks, and the treatment is then stopped finally.

- For some patients, the disease relapses soon after the treatment is terminated, or alternative treatment modalities are not available or contraindicated. In such cases, once per fortnight maintenance therapy may be continued for several weeks or even months to keep the skin disease under control.
- The following table shows a general guideline for combined UVA/NBUVB dosimetry in these situations.

Tapered Frequency of Treatment	Dose Adjustment
Once per week	Hold dose
Once every two weeks (up to 12 months)	↓ dose by 25% of previous dose and hold

Further Reading

1. Fernández-Guarino M, Aboin-Gonzalez S, Barchino L, *et al.* Treatment of moderate and severe adult chronic atopic dermatitis with narrow-band UVB and the combination of narrow-band UVB/UVA phototherapy. *Dermatol Ther* 2016; 29: 19–23.
2. Jekler J, Larkö O. Combined UVA-UVB versus UVB phototherapy for atopic dermatitis: A paired-comparison study. *J Am Acad Dermatol* 1990; 22: 49–53.
3. Jekler J, Larkö O. Phototherapy for atopic dermatitis with ultraviolet A (UVA), low-dose UVB and combined UVA and UVB: Two paired-comparison studies. *Photodermatol Photoimmunol Photomed* 1991; 8: 151–156.
4. Koh MJ, Chong WS. Aquagenic pruritus responding to combined ultraviolet A/narrowband ultraviolet B therapy. *Photodermatol Photoimmunol Photomed* 2009; 25: 169–170.

5. Macias VC, Marques-Pinto G, Cardoso J. Phototherapy for pityriasis lichenoides: Our experience. *Cutan Ocul Toxicol* 2013; 32: 124–127.
6. Meduri NB, Vandergriff T, Rasmussen H, *et al.* Phototherapy in the management of atopic dermatitis: A systematic review. *Photodermatol Photoimmunol Photomed* 2007; 23: 106–112.
7. Midelfart K, Stenvold SE, Volden G. Combined UVB and UVA phototherapy of atopic eczema. *Dermatologica* 1985; 171: 95–98.
8. Valkova S, Velkova A. UVA/UVB phototherapy for atopic dermatitis revisited. *J Dermatolog Treat* 2004; 5: 239–244.

Chapter

5

Psoralen-Ultraviolet A Photochemotherapy

Background

- Psoralen-ultraviolet A (PUVA) photochemotherapy refers to the combined use of psoralen and UVA radiation. This drug-radiation combination produces a therapeutic effect that is not achieved by the single component alone. Repeated controlled phototoxic reactions result in the remission of the dermatoses.
- Due to a higher risk of treatment-related skin cancers, the use of PUVA photochemotherapy has declined in recent years in favour of narrowband UVB (NBUVB) phototherapy. Nevertheless, it

remains a useful treatment modality in certain dermatoses, and in recalcitrant diseases not responding to NBUVB phototherapy.

PUVA Modalities: Practical Aspects

Psoralen may be delivered to the skin in a few ways.

Oral PUVA Photochemotherapy

- 8-methoxypsoralen (8-MOP) or methoxsalen is given orally, at a dose of 0.4 to 0.6 mg/kg body weight. If Meladinine® (CLS Pharma) is used as 8-MOP, the drug is taken two hours (not later than three hours) before UVA irradiation, using the whole-body UVA unit.
- The most commonly reported side effect of 8-MOP alone is nausea, which occurs with approximately 10% of all patients. This effect may be minimised or avoided by instructing the patient to take the drug with a light meal comprising low-fat food, with or without milk, and/or to divide the dose into two portions, taken 30 minutes apart. It is important to ensure consistency in the type and quantity of food consumed each time. This is to ensure consistent peak serum drug level and consistent time of peak photosensitivity before each irradiation.

Bath/Soak PUVA Photochemotherapy

- In bath PUVA photochemotherapy, the patient is bathed in warm water with 8-MOP solution added to a final concentration of 3.75 mg/L at 37°C, by diluting 60 mL of 0.75% 8-MOP solution (Meladinine®, CLS Pharma) in a total final volume of 120 L of water.
- Soak PUVA photochemotherapy is used to treat dermatoses involving hands and/or feet. In this technique, the patient's hands and/or feet are soaked in water with 8-MOP solution added to a final concentration of 3.75 mg/L, by diluting 1–2 mL of 0.75% 8-MOP solution (Meladinine®, CLS Pharma) in a total final volume of 2–4 L of water (Figure 2).

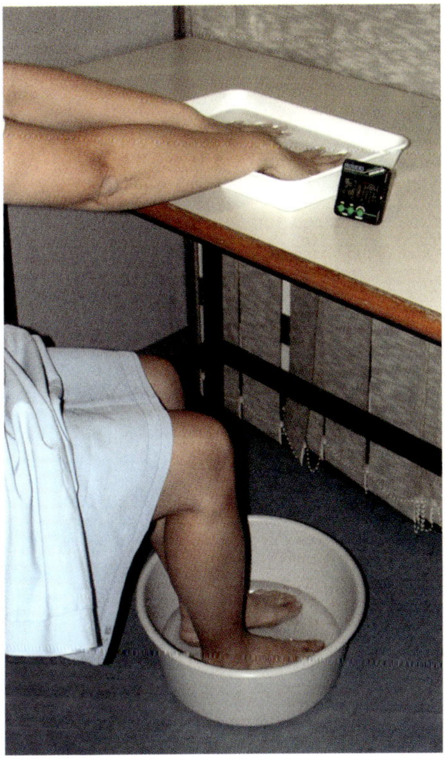

Figure 2. In soak PUVA photochemotherapy, the hands and feet are soaked in 8-MOP solution prior to UVA irradiation.

- The bath/soak time is 20 minutes, after which the patient is exposed to UVA radiation immediately, or within 15 minutes. The whole-body UVA unit is utilised in bath PUVA photochemotherapy, whereas the localised hand/foot UVA units (both curved-panel and flat-panel) are used in soak PUVA photochemotherapy.
- When treating lesions on the legs, a special form of soak PUVA known as barrel PUVA can be utilised. In this technique, each leg is soaked in water with 8-MOP solution added to a final concentration of 3.75 mg/L, by diluting 2.5–12 mL of 0.75% 8-MOP solution (Meladinine®, CLS Pharma) in a total final volume of 5–24 L of water. After a soak time of 20 minutes, each leg is then placed

in turn at the centre of a barrel configuration formed by two curved-panel UVA units placed together (Figure 3).

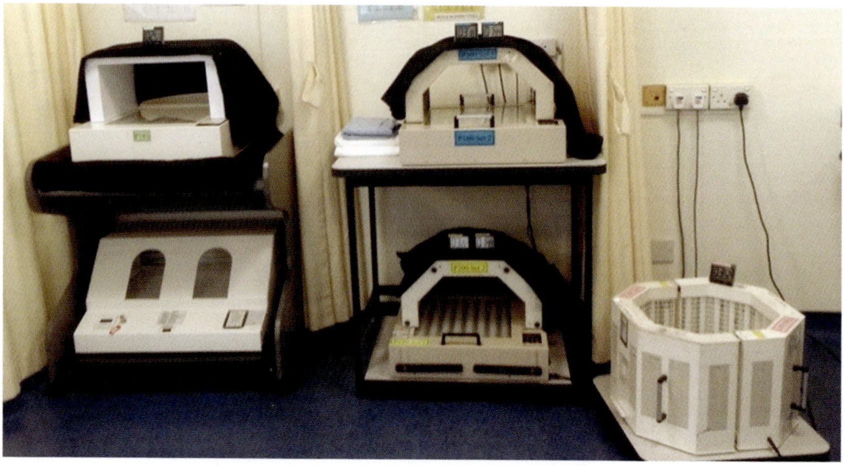

Figure 3. Localised curved-panel and flat-panel UVA units for soak and barrel PUVA photochemotherapies.

- Advantages of bath and soak PUVA photochemotherapies include the avoidance of systemic side effects and ocular toxicity due to oral 8-MOP. The barrel PUVA technique obviates the need to cover the whole body while irradiating the legs in the whole-body cabin (as in bath PUVA), thus avoiding unnecessary exposure of UVA to the rest of the body that is not treated.

Paint PUVA Photochemotherapy

- In paint PUVA photochemotherapy, 0.1% 8-MOP solution (Meladinine®, CLS Pharma) is applied as a thin layer with a cotton swab to lesional skin, taking care to avoid applying to surrounding unaffected skin. There is a waiting time of 20 minutes before UVA irradiation. The flat-panel UVA canopy unit is utilised in paint PUVA photochemotherapy.
- When treating scalp lesions such as alopecia areata in scalp PUVA, the curved-panel UVA unit is used in combination with a flat-panel UVA unit; the former is positioned above the head and the latter is positioned behind the head.

- When treating very sensitive and thin skin areas, the 8-MOP solution may be further diluted to 0.01% if necessary.
- Once a maximum dose of 5 J/cm^2 is reached, the 8-MOP solution of higher strength such as 0.75% 8-MOP may be used, with the UVA dose reduced appropriately to avoid a PUVA burn.

Paint PUVASol

- Vitiligo is one of the dermatoses most commonly treated using the paint PUVASol technique.
- The patient is instructed to apply 0.1% 8-MOP solution (Meladinine®, CLS Pharma) thinly using a cotton swab to lesional skin, and wait for a further 20 minutes before solar exposure.
- The lesional skin is exposed to sunlight at the same time of the day at every treatment session, either in the early morning before 11 a.m. or late afternoon after 3 p.m.
- Treatment is performed twice per week on non-consecutive days, every 3–4 days apart.
- Solar exposure times are increased very gradually, on a weekly basis, beginning with 15 seconds in the first week, then followed by 30 seconds in the second week. From the third week onwards, the exposure time is increased by 30 seconds every week, until a maximum of 60 minutes if the erythema caused by the treatment is not excessive.
- The objective is to achieve an asymptomatic, faint erythema on the treated skin. When an asymptomatic, faint erythema is achieved, treatment time is kept constant.
- After each treatment, the 8-MOP solution is immediately washed off thoroughly. The patient should minimise further exposure to the sun by wearing a long-sleeved shirt with long pants (depending on the extent and location of the treated skin) or by carrying an umbrella when going outdoors, and by applying a sunscreen.

Indications of PUVA Photochemotherapy

- PUVA photochemotherapy is usually utilised as second-line treatment after failure of NBUVB phototherapy.
- To avoid systemic side effects due to oral 8-MOP, the PUVA modality usually employed is either bath, soak or paint PUVA, depending on the clinical problem. However, in mycosis fungoides, oral PUVA is the modality of choice.

Common

- Psoriasis [A, Ia]
- Palmoplantar psoriasis/pustulosis [A, Ib]
- Hand/foot eczema [A, Ib]
- Mycosis fungoides [B, IIa]

Less Common

- Alopecia areata [B, III]
- Vitiligo
  - Oral/bath/paint PUVA [A, Ib]
  - Topical PUVASol [B, III]
- Atopic dermatitis [A, Ib]
- Pityriasis lichenoides [A, Ib]

Contraindications to PUVA Photochemotherapy

Absolute

- Severe medical illness that prevents standing in the phototherapy cabin (oral/bath PUVA)
- Haemodynamic instability
- Systemic lupus erythematosus, dermatomyositis
- Genophotodermatoses (e.g. xeroderma pigmentosum)
- Photosensitivity
- Personal history of melanoma

Relative

- Personal history of non-melanoma skin cancer (NMSC)
- Pre-malignant skin lesions (e.g. actinic keratosis)

- Atypical naevus syndrome
- Family history of skin cancer
- Previous exposure to arsenic or ionising radiation
- Poorly controlled epilepsy
- Photosensitising drugs
- Treatment with immunosuppressive drugs that significantly increase the risk of skin cancer (e.g. ciclosporin)

Due to Oral 8-MOP

- Pregnancy — 8-MOP is under pregnancy category C
- Breastfeeding — can only commence 24 hours after oral 8-MOP ingestion
- Cataract
- Significant hepatic and renal dysfunction
- Children younger than 12 years old

Adverse Effects of PUVA Photochemotherapy

Acute

- Pruritus (PUVA itch)
- Pain (PUVA pain)
- Erythema
- Blistering
- Pigmentation (Tanning)
- Melanonychia
- Photo-onycholysis
- Hypertrichosis
- Aggravation of existing skin disease
- Provocation of polymorphic light eruption (PMLE)

Due to Oral 8-MOP

- Nausea, abdominal discomfort, epigastric pain
- Headache, dizziness, insomnia, hyperactivity, depression
- Generalised malaise
- Exanthem, drug fever
- Bronchoconstriction

- Hepatotoxicity
- Ocular phototoxicity
- Drug interactions e.g. photosensitising drugs, cytochrome P450 enzyme inducers/inhibitors, warfarin

Chronic

- Premature photoageing
- PUVA lentigines and keratoses
- Skin malignancy, especially squamous cell carcinoma (SCC)

Screening and Monitoring (Oral PUVA Photochemotherapy)

- Patients should undergo an ophthalmologic examination prior to the start of oral PUVA photochemotherapy, and annually thereafter.

- Patients should have routine hepatic and renal function tests done prior to the start of oral PUVA photochemotherapy, and at regular periods thereafter if patients are on extended treatments. The frequency of repeat blood tests would be suggested by findings of history or examination.

Treatment Regimen and Dosimetry

Treatment Initiation

- PUVA photochemotherapy is started at a frequency of two to three times per week.

- The objective is to deliver a suberythemogenic dose of UVA to achieve the best therapeutic response. The initial UVA dose (J/cm^2) can be determined by one of two approaches:

Approach #1: MPD Regimen [A, Ib]

- The patient's minimal phototoxic dose (MPD) is determined prior to commencing PUVA photochemotherapy. The MPD regimen is individually tailored and considered to be the safest and most optimal dosimetry for the patient.

- We routinely use 70% of MPD as the initial UVA dose for oral PUVA, and 30% of MPD as the initial dose for bath PUVA as bath PUVA photochemotherapy is ten times more phototoxic than oral PUVA photochemotherapy. Refer to Chapter 9 — Phototesting and Annex B for details of MPD testing and the dosimetry respectively.

Oral PUVA: Initial UVA dose = 70% of MPD
Bath PUVA: Initial UVA dose = 30% of MPD

Approach #2: Skin Phototype Regimen [C, IV]

- This method, based on skin phototype, is generally used in a patient whose skin disease is so extensive that there is inadequate normal skin for MPD testing.
- In practice, this method is more convenient and preferred in some busy phototherapy centres with a heavy patient load as it may be impractical to conduct MPD testing for every patient.
- In soak PUVA and paint PUVA photochemotherapies, only the skin phototype regimen is utilised for practical reasons.
- The following tables illustrate the starting dosimetry for oral, bath, soak and paint PUVA photochemotherapies.

Oral PUVA Starting Dosimetry

Skin Phototype	**Initial UVA Dose (J/cm²)**
I	0.5
II	1.0
III	1.5
IV	2.0
V	2.5
VI	3.0

Bath PUVA Starting Dosimetry

Skin Phototype	Initial UVA Dose (J/cm^2)
I	0.3
II	0.4
III	0.5
IV	0.6
V	0.7
VI	0.8

Soak/Paint PUVA Starting Dosimetry

Skin	Initial UVA Dose (J/cm^2)	
Phototype	Dorsum/Flat/Thin	Palm/Sole/Thick
I	0.25	0.5
II	0.25	0.5
III	0.5	0.75
IV	0.5	0.75
V	0.75	1.0
VI	0.75	1.0

Dose Adjustment Based on Erythema [C, IV]

- The goal of photochemotherapy is to maintain a mild, just perceptible erythema throughout the treatment course.
- On each subsequent visit, the patient's severity of erythema is assessed in order to determine the dose adjustment (as shown in the following table). Depending on the erythema response, the dose of UVA is usually increased with each session to counteract the effects of photoadaptation due to the photochemotherapy, namely epidermal hyperplasia and pigmentation (tanning).

Oral PUVA Dose Adjustment

Erythema History	Erythema Grading	Description of Erythema on Attendance	Dose Adjustment
None	0	No erythema	↑ by 20% of MPD or 1 J/cm^2
< 7 days	±	No erythema (erythema is reported only by patient)	↑ by 10% of MPD or 0.5 J/cm^2
7–9 days	+	Just perceptible pink erythema, asymptomatic	Hold dose
≥ 7–9 days	++	Well-defined erythema, possibly causing slight manageable discomfort	↓ by 25% of previous dose, or postpone treatment. When settled, restart after three days at previous dose.
Painful without blistering	+++	Well-defined fiery-red erythema, symptomatic, painful	No treatment. Review by doctor. When settled, restart after one week at 50% of previous dose.
Painful with blistering	++++	Well-defined fiery-red, painful erythema with blistering	No treatment. Review by doctor. When settled, restart after one week at 50% of previous dose.

Bath/Soak/Paint PUVA Dose Adjustment

Erythema History	Erythema Grading	Description of Erythema on Attendance	Dose Adjustment
None	0	No erythema	↑ by 20% of MPD or 0.5 J/cm^2
< 7 days	±	No erythema (erythema is reported only by patient)	↑ by 10% of MPD or 0.25 J/cm^2

(*Continued*)

Table (*Continued*)

Erythema History	Erythema Grading	Description of Erythema on Attendance	Dose Adjustment
7-9 days	+	Just perceptible pink erythema, asymptomatic	Hold dose
≥ 7-9 days	++	Well-defined erythema, possibly causing slight manageable discomfort	↓ by 25% of previous dose, or postpone treatment. When settled, restart after three days at previous dose.
Painful without blistering	+++	Well-defined fiery-red erythema, symptomatic, painful	No treatment. Review by doctor. When settled, restart after one week at 50% of previous dose.
Painful with blistering	++++	Well-defined fiery-red, painful erythema with blistering	No treatment. Review by doctor. When settled, restart after one week at 50% of previous dose.

- If lesions on the lower legs and feet appear slow to respond, give them an additional 20% to 30% of the total body dose, with the rest of the body covered, and the patient standing on a platform of 12 to 16-cm height.

Paint PUVA Photochemotherapy for Psoriasis [C, IV]

- The dosimetry is based on both skin phototype and plaque induration/thickness.
- Refer to the earlier part of this section on the starting dosimetry for paint PUVA photochemotherapy.
- On each subsequent visit, the patient's severity of erythema and degree of plaque improvement (denoted as plaque quality) are assessed in order to determine the dose adjustment (as shown

in the following table). Depending on the plaque quality, the UVA dose is usually increased with each session to counteract the effects of photoadaptation due to the photochemotherapy, namely epidermal hyperplasia and pigmentation (tanning).

Erythema History	**Erythema Grading**	**Plaque Quality on Attendance**	**Dose Adjustment**
None	0	No erythema, no plaque improvement, no pigmentation	↑ by 0.5 J/cm^2
< 7 days	±	No erythema (erythema is reported only by patient), minimal plaque improvement, minimal pigmentation	↑ by 0.25 J/cm^2
7–9 days	+	Mild erythema, plaque thinning, reduced scaliness, pigmentation present	Hold dose
≥ 7–9 days	++	Moderate erythema, possibly causing slight manageable discomfort	↓ by 25% of previous dose, or postpone treatment. When settled, restart after three days at previous dose.
Painful without blistering	+++	Fiery-red erythema, symptomatic, painful	No treatment. Review by doctor. When settled, restart after one week at 50% of previous dose.
Painful with blistering	++++	Fiery-red, painful erythema with blistering	No treatment. Review by doctor. When settled, restart after one week at 50% of previous dose.

Maximum Dose per Session based on Skin Phototype [C, IV]

- The maximum UVA dose delivered per session should not be exceeded unless otherwise considered, as shown in the table below.

Skin Phototype	Maximum UVA Dose (J/cm^2)
I	10
II	10
III	15
IV	15
V	20
VI	20

Missed Treatment Protocol [C, IV]

- If a patient's treatment is missed or cancelled, the UVA dose should be adjusted accordingly as shown in the table below, based on the treatment interval between the previous and current sessions. In a situation when treatment is omitted due to erythema, the dose adjustment protocol based on erythema should be followed instead.

Treatment Interval (days)	Dose Adjustment
1 to 7	Hold dose or ↑ dose as per protocol
8 to 14	↓ dose by 25% of previous dose
15 to 21	↓ dose by 50% of previous dose
22 to 28	↓ dose by 75% of previous dose
> 28	Refer back to doctor, start over

Maintenance Therapy [C, IV]

- After the skin lesions have cleared or markedly improved (e.g. > 75% improvement), the patient may be continued on maintenance therapy to prevent a relapse of the disease. If the patient has started PUVA photochemotherapy three times per week during the clearing phase of treatment, depending on the response, the frequency of treatment sessions may be gradually reduced to two times per week for several weeks, followed by once per week for several weeks, and the treatment is then stopped finally.

- For some patients, the disease relapses soon after the treatment is terminated, or alternative treatment modalities are not available or contraindicated. In such cases, once per fortnight maintenance therapy may be continued for several weeks or even months to keep the skin disease under control.
- The following table shows a general guideline to PUVA dosimetry in these situations.

Tapered Frequency of Treatment	Dose Adjustment
Once per week	Hold dose
Once every two weeks (up to 12 months)	↓ dose by 25% of previous dose and hold

Retinoid-PUVA (Re-PUVA) Treatment Regimen and Dosimetry [C, IV]

- The combination of a systemic retinoid such as acitretin and PUVA photochemotherapy is best done using the MPD regimen, in the case of oral and bath PUVA photochemotherapies. In Re-PUVA photochemotherapy, the initiation of the retinoid therapy should be done prior to the commencement of PUVA treatment. In this case, the retinoid is initiated for a period of two weeks before performing UVA phototesting to determine the MPD-Re-PUVA. Obtaining the MPD at this time gives a more accurate and effective dose of UVA and prevents phototoxic reactions from the treatment.
- However, when phototesting to determine MPD-Re-PUVA is not feasible, skin phototype regimen is then used with the starting

dose of UVA equivalent to 50% of the original initial UVA dose based on the respective skin phototype.

- In the case when the systemic retinoid is started after the patient has already undergone induction of PUVA photochemotherapy, the dose of UVA is maintained for a period of two weeks after the introduction of the retinoid, followed by subsequent dose adjustment based on the erythema response.

Skin Cancer Surveillance for Patients on Long-Term PUVA Photochemotherapy [C, IV]

- As with other phototherapies, there is no clear-cut evidence on which to base a recommendation for a maximum lifetime number of treatments.
- Patients receiving more than 250 PUVA treatment sessions should be considered as possibly being at increased risk of skin cancer and managed accordingly with regular skin cancer surveillance and close monitoring for skin malignancy.

Further Reading

1. Archier E, Devaux S, Castela E, *et al.* Carcinogenic risks of psoralen UV-A therapy and narrowband UV-B therapy in chronic plaque psoriasis: A systematic literature review. *J Eur Acad Dermatol Venereol* 2012; 26: 22–31.
2. Archier E, Devaux S, Castela E, *et al.* Efficacy of psoralen UV-A therapy vs. narrowband UV-B therapy in chronic plaque psoriasis: A systematic literature review. *J Eur Acad Dermatol Venereol* 2012; 26: 11–21.
3. Handa S, Pandhi R, Kaur I. Vitiligo: A retrospective comparative analysis of treatment modalities in 500 patients. *J Dermatol* 2001; 28: 461–466.
4. Henseler T, Wolff K, Hönigsmann H, *et al.* Oral 8-methoxypsoralen photochemotherapy of psoriasis, the European PUVA study: A cooperative study among 18 European centers. *Lancet* 1981; 1: 853–857.
5. Krutman J, Hoenigsmann H, Elmets CA. *Dermatological Phototherapy and Photodiagnostic Methods,* 2nd ed. Berlin, Heidelberg: Springer-Verlag; 2009.

6. Melski JW, Tanenbaum L, Parrish JA, *et al*. Oral methoxsalen photochemotherapy for the treatment of psoriasis: A cooperative clinical trial. *J Invest Dermatol* 1977; 68: 328–335.
7. Sezer E, Erbil AH, Kurumlu Z, *et al*. Comparison of the efficacy of local narrowband ultraviolet B (NB-UVB) phototherapy versus psoralen plus ultraviolet A (PUVA) paint for palmoplantar psoriasis. *J Dermatol* 2007; 34: 435–440.
8. Zanolli MD, Feldman SR. *Phototherapy Treatment Protocols for Psoriasis and Other Phototherapy-Responsive Dermatoses,* 2nd ed. New York: Taylor & Francis Group; 2004.

Chapter

6

Ultraviolet A-1 Phototherapy

Background

- Lamps emitting UVR in the 340–400 nm (UVA-1) spectrum have various therapeutic uses.
- UVA-1 radiation reduces cutaneous inflammatory cells such as T lymphocytes, Langerhans cells and dermal mast cells via apoptosis, and induces matrix metalloproteinase production by fibroblasts.

Delivery of UVA-1

- UVA-1 may be delivered as localised or whole-body treatment (Figure 4). However, due to the large amount of heat produced

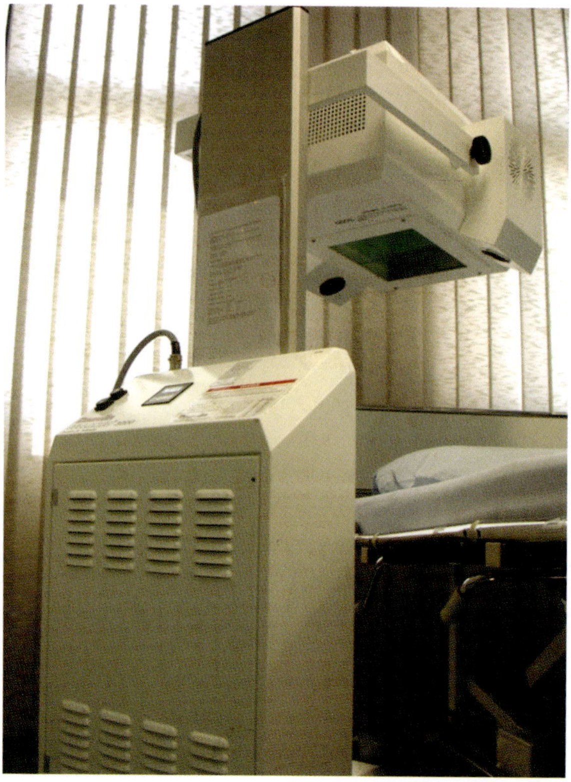

Figure 4. Localised flat-panel UVA-1 phototherapy unit.

especially when delivering UVA-1 in medium and high doses, whole-body treatment units utilising high-output metal halide lamps require elaborate cooling systems, and are not widely available.

- Other limitations to the use of UVA-1 phototherapy include large amount of heat produced when delivering UVA-1 in medium and high doses causing discomfort to the patient, long irradiation time and high cost of the equipment that houses the high-output metal halide lamp.

Indications of UVA-1 Phototherapy

Common

• Hand and/or foot eczema	[A, Ib]
• Localised scleroderma/Morphoea	[A, Ib]
• Graft-versus-host disease	[B, III]

Less common

• Atopic dermatitis	[A, Ib]
• Lichen sclerosus	[B, III]
• Systemic sclerosis	[B, III]
• Scleroedema	[B, III]
• Granuloma annulare	[B, III]
• Necrobiosis lipoidica	[B, III]
• Cutaneous mastocytosis	[B, III]
• Cutaneous T-cell lymphoma	[B, III]
• Systemic lupus erythematosus	[B, IIa]

Contraindications to UVA-1 Phototherapy

Absolute

- Severe medical illness that prevents standing in the phototherapy cabin (whole-body standing unit)
- Haemodynamic instability (whole-body standing unit)
- Genophotodermatoses (e.g. xeroderma pigmentosum)
- Photosensitivity
- Personal history of melanoma

Relative

- Personal history of non-melanoma skin cancer (NMSC)
- Pre-malignant skin lesions (e.g. actinic keratosis)
- Atypical naevus syndrome
- Family history of skin cancer
- Previous exposure to arsenic or ionising radiation

- Poorly controlled epilepsy (whole-body standing unit)
- Photosensitising drugs
- Treatment with immunosuppressive drugs that significantly increase the risk of skin cancer (e.g. ciclosporin)

Adverse Effects of UVA-1 Phototherapy

Acute

- Pigmentation (Tanning)
- Pruritus
- Erythema
- Aggravation of existing skin disease
- Provocation of polymorphic light eruption (PMLE)

Chronic

- Premature photoageing
- Skin malignancy, especially squamous cell carcinoma (SCC)

Dosimetry Regimens

- While the dosimetry regimens are not standardised internationally, the following definitions of low, medium and high target doses of UVA-1 are generally acceptable.

UVA-1 Regimen	Target Dose
Low dose	20 J/cm^2
Medium dose	60 J/cm^2
High dose	130 J/cm^2

- The UVA-1 dosimetry schedule is as follows:
  - UVA-1 phototherapy is started at a frequency of three to five times per week.
  - Initial dose of UVA-1 is 20 J/cm^2.
  - Assess prior to starting the next treatment session.

- If no adverse effect such as erythema, pruritus, desquamation or burning sensation occurs after the last treatment, the subsequent UVA-1 dose may be adjusted according to the regimen considered. The high-dose UVA-1 regimen is the preferred regimen unless otherwise considered.

UVA-1 Regimen	Dose Adjustment
Low dose	Hold dose at 20 J/cm^2
Medium dose	↑ by 10 J/cm^2 till 60 J/cm^2
High dose	↑ by 10 J/cm^2 till 130 J/cm^2

- If adverse effects such as erythema, pruritus, desquamation or burning sensation occur after the last treatment, the subsequent UVA-1 dose may be adjusted according to the following table.

Adverse Effect	Dose Adjustment
Mild	Hold dose
Moderate	↓ by 25% of previous dose, or postpone treatment. When settled, restart after three days at previous dose.
Severe	No treatment. Review by doctor. When settled, restart after one week at 50% of previous dose.

Missed Treatment Protocol [C, IV]

- If a patient's treatment is missed or cancelled, the UVA-1 dose should be adjusted accordingly as shown in the table below, based on the treatment interval between the previous and current sessions.

Treatment Interval (days)	Dose Adjustment
1 to 7	Hold dose or ↑ dose as per protocol
8 to 14	↓ dose by 25% of previous dose
15 to 21	↓ dose by 50% of previous dose
22 to 28	↓ dose by 75% of previous dose
> 28	Refer back to doctor, start over

Maintenance Therapy [C, IV]

- After the skin lesions have cleared or markedly improved (e.g. > 75% improvement), the patient may be continued on maintenance therapy to prevent a relapse of the disease. If the patient has started UVA-1 phototherapy three to five times per week during the clearing phase of treatment, depending on the response, the frequency of treatment sessions may be gradually reduced to two times per week for several weeks, followed by once per week for several weeks, and the treatment is then stopped finally.
- For some patients, the disease relapses soon after the treatment is terminated, or alternative treatment modalities are not available or contraindicated. In such cases, once per fortnight maintenance therapy may be continued for several weeks or even months to keep the skin disease under control.
- The following table shows a general guideline for UVA-1 dosimetry in these situations.

Tapered Frequency of Treatment	Dose Adjustment
Once per week	Hold dose
Once every two weeks (up to 12 months)	↓ dose by 25% of previous dose and hold

Skin Cancer Surveillance for Patients on Long-Term UVA-1 Phototherapy [C, IV]

- As with other phototherapies, there is no clear-cut evidence on which to base a recommendation for a maximum lifetime number of treatments.
- Patients receiving > 250 UVA-1 treatment sessions should be considered as possibly being at increased risk of skin cancer and managed accordingly with regular skin cancer surveillance and close monitoring for skin malignancy.

Further Reading

1. Kerr AC, Ferguson J, Attili SK, *et al*. Ultraviolet A1 phototherapy: A British Photodermatology Group workshop report. *Clin Exp Dermatol* 2012; 37: 219–226.
2. Kreuter A, Hyun J, Stücker M, *et al*. A randomized controlled study of low-dose UVA1, medium-dose UVA1, and narrowband UVB phototherapy in the treatment of localized scleroderma. *J Am Acad Dermatol* 2006; 54: 440–447.
3. Polderman MCA, Govaert JCM, le Cessie S, *et al*. A double-blind placebo-controlled trial of UVA1 in the treatment of dyshidrotic eczema. *Clin Exp Dermatol* 2003; 28: 584–587.
4. Schmidt T, Abeck D, Seitzer U, *et al*. UVA1 irradiation is effective in treatment of chronic vesicular dyshidrotic hand eczema. *Acta Derm Venereol* 1998; 78: 318–319.
5. Stege H, Berneburg M, Humke S, *et al*. High-dose UVA1 radiation therapy for localized scleroderma. *J Am Acad Dermatol* 1997; 36: 938–944.

Chapter

7

Excimer Light Phototherapy

Background

- Targeted phototherapy refers to the use of light or laser of a specific wavelength targeting localised lesional skin only, usually covering body surface area (BSA) of less than 5%, via special delivery mechanisms.
- The objective is to use the highest possible light or laser dose to clear the lesion in the shortest possible time.
- Potential advantages over conventional phototherapy include the following:
    - Ability to use higher doses on affected skin only.
    - Faster clinical response with fewer treatment sessions.

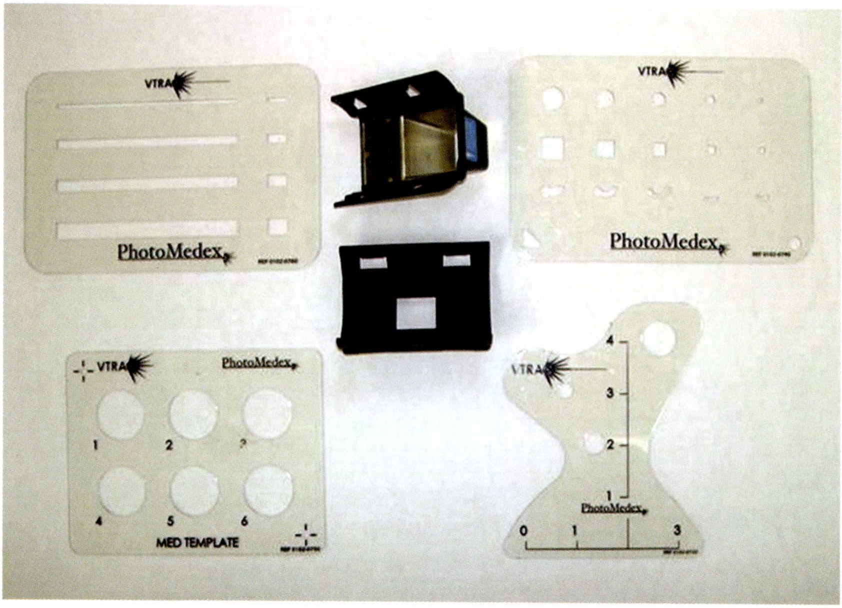

Figure 5. Transparent templates and black lamp apertures applied onto the skin are used to facilitate targeted irradiation during excimer light phototherapy.

- ○ Sparing uninvolved skin from UVR, thereby avoiding side effects such as erythema, pigmentation (tanning) and premature skin ageing on these sites (Figure 5).
- ○ Lower total cumulative UVR dose.
- ○ Ability to target covered anatomical sites or sanctuary sites (e.g. scalp, axillae, gluteal cleft and inguinal regions).
- ○ Less bulky equipment.

- The most common targeted phototherapy devices include the 308-nm excimer laser system, 308-nm excimer lamp system and other non-excimer light systems which can be office or home-based. The most widely studied of all these systems are the excimer light devices (Figure 6).

Excimer Light

- Both excimer laser and excimer lamp systems emit excimer light.

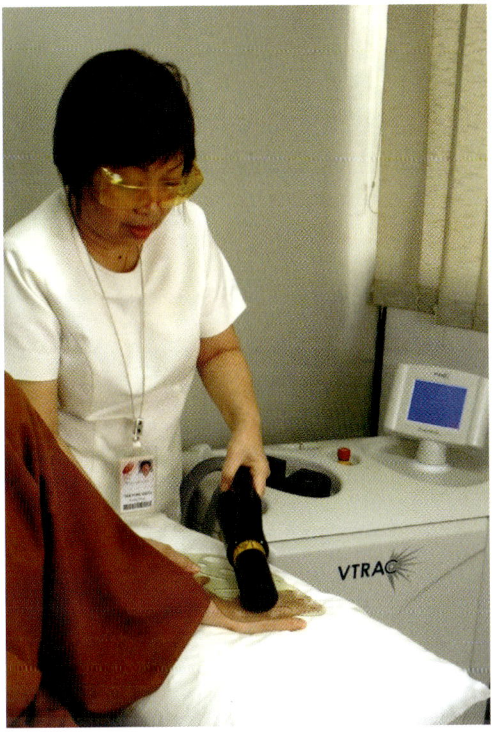

Figure 6. Targeted UVB phototherapy with excimer light device.

- The excimer laser system produces monochromatic coherent light at 308 nm, while the excimer lamp system produces polychromatic incoherent light at 308 ± 2 nm.

Indications of Excimer Light Phototherapy [B, IIA]

- Stable localised or recalcitrant plaque psoriasis, with BSA < 5% involvement
- Vitiligo, with BSA < 5% involvement
- Difficult covered anatomical sites or sanctuary sites such as scalp, axillae, gluteal cleft, inguinal regions and skin folds
- Other dermatoses responsive to NBUVB, with BSA < 5% involvement
- Children who are claustrophobic in the NBUVB phototherapy cabin

Contraindications to Excimer Light Phototherapy

Absolute

- Systemic lupus erythematosus, dermatomyositis
- Genophotodermatoses (e.g. xeroderma pigmentosum)
- Photosensitivity
- Personal history of melanoma

Relative

- Personal history of non-melanoma skin cancer (NMSC)
- Pre-malignant skin lesions (e.g. actinic keratosis)
- Atypical naevus syndrome
- Family history of skin cancer
- Previous exposure to arsenic or ionising radiation
- Photosensitising drugs
- Treatment with immunosuppressive drugs that significantly increase the risk of skin cancer (e.g. ciclosporin)

Adverse Effects of Excimer Light Phototherapy

Acute

- Erythema
- Blistering
- Pain
- Pruritus
- Pigmentation (Tanning)
- Aggravation of existing skin disease
- Koebner phenomenon
- Herpes simplex virus reactivation
- Corneal burn

Chronic

- Premature photoageing
- Skin malignancy, especially squamous cell carcinoma (SCC)

Psoriasis Protocol [C, IV]

- Evidence-based studies on excimer light dosimetry for the treatment of psoriasis are limited, and there is no standardised protocol currently.
- Treatment is initiated at a frequency of two to three times per week.
- The dosimetry is based on both skin phototype and plaque induration/thickness.
- The initial dose and subsequent dose increment schedules are illustrated in the following two tables.

Skin Phototype	Initial Dose (mJ/cm^2)		
	Flat/Thin	**Medium Thick**	**Very Thick**
I	100	200	300
II	150	300	450
III	200	400	600
IV	250	500	750
V	300	600	900
VI	350	700	1050

Skin Phototype	Dose Increment (mJ/cm^2)	
	Full Dose	**Half Dose**
I	50	25
II	75	37
III	100	50
IV	125	62
V	150	75
VI	175	87

Dose Adjustment Based on Erythema and Plaque Improvement = Plaque Quality [C, IV]

- On each subsequent visit, the patient's severity of erythema and degree of plaque improvement (denoted as plaque quality) are assessed in order to determine the dose adjustment (as shown in the following table). Depending on the plaque quality, the excimer light dose is usually increased with each session to counteract the effects of photoadaptation due to the phototherapy, namely epidermal hyperplasia and pigmentation (tanning).

Erythema History	Erythema Grading	Plaque Quality on Attendance	Dose Adjustment
None	0	No erythema, no plaque improvement, no pigmentation	↑ by full dose
< 48 hours	±	No erythema (erythema is reported only by patient), minimal plaque improvement, minimal pigmentation	↑ by half dose
48–72 hours	+	Mild erythema, plaque thinning, reduced scaliness, pigmentation present	Hold dose
≥ 48–72 hours	++	Moderate erythema, possibly causing slight manageable discomfort	↓ by 25% of previous dose, or postpone treatment. When settled, restart after three days at previous dose.
Painful without blistering	+++	Fiery-red erythema, symptomatic, painful	No treatment. Review by doctor. When settled, restart after one week at 50% of previous dose.
Painful with blistering	++++	Fiery-red, painful erythema with blistering	No treatment. Review by doctor. When settled, restart after one week at 50% of previous dose.

Maximum Dose per Session based on Skin Phototype [C, IV]

- The maximum excimer light dose delivered per session should not be exceeded unless otherwise considered, as shown in the table below.

Skin Phototype	**Maximum Dose (mJ/cm²)**
I	4000
II	4000
III	5000
IV	5000
V	6000
VI	6000

Missed Treatment Protocol [C, IV]

- If a patient's treatment is missed or cancelled, the excimer light dose should be adjusted accordingly as shown in the table below, based on the treatment interval between the previous and current sessions. In a situation when treatment is omitted due to erythema, the dose adjustment protocol based on erythema should be followed instead.

Treatment Interval (days)	**Dose Adjustment**
1 to 7	Hold dose or ↑ dose as per protocol
8 to 14	↓ dose by 25% of previous dose
15 to 21	↓ dose by 50% of previous dose
22 to 28	↓ dose by 75% of previous dose
> 28	Refer back to doctor, start over

Vitiligo Protocol [C, IV]

- Evidence-based studies on excimer light dosimetry for the treatment of vitiligo are limited, and there is no standardised protocol currently.

- Treatment is initiated at a frequency of two to three times per week.
- The dosimetry is based on skin phototype I.

Skin Phototype	Dose (mJ/cm²) Initial Dose	Full Dose Increment	Half Dose Increment
I	100	50	25

Dose Adjustment Based on Erythema [C, IV]

- The goal of phototherapy is to maintain a mild, just perceptible erythema throughout the treatment course.
- On each subsequent visit, the patient's severity of erythema is assessed in order to determine the dose adjustment (as shown in the following table). Depending on the erythema response, the excimer light dose is usually increased with each session to

Erythema History	Erythema Grading	Description of Erythema on Attendance	Dose Adjustment
None	0	No erythema	↑ by full dose
< 48 hours	±	No erythema (erythema is reported only by patient)	↑ by half dose
48–72 hours	+	Just perceptible pink erythema, asymptomatic	Hold dose
≥ 48–72 hours	++	Well-defined erythema, possibly causing slight manageable discomfort	↓ by 25% of previous dose, or postpone treatment. When settled, restart after three days at previous dose.

(Continued)

Table *(Continued)*

Erythema History	Erythema Grading	Description of Erythema on Attendance	Dose Adjustment
Painful without blistering	+++	Well-defined fiery-red erythema, symptomatic, painful	No treatment. Review by doctor. When settled, restart after one week at 50% of previous dose.
Painful with blistering	++++	Well-defined fiery-red, painful erythema with blistering	No treatment. Review by doctor. When settled, restart after one week at 50% of previous dose.

counteract the effects of photoadaptation due to the phototherapy, namely epidermal hyperplasia and pigmentation (tanning).

Maximum Dose per Session based on Skin Phototype [C, IV]

- The maximum excimer light dose delivered per session should not be exceeded unless otherwise considered, as shown in the table below. This maximum dose is based on the patient's constitutional skin phototype.

Skin Phototype	Maximum Dose (mJ/cm^2)
I	4000
II	4000
III	5000
IV	5000
V	6000
VI	6000

Missed Treatment Protocol [C, IV]

- If a patient's treatment is missed or cancelled, the excimer light dose should be adjusted accordingly as shown in the table below, based on the treatment interval between the previous and current sessions. In a situation when treatment is omitted due to erythema, the dose adjustment protocol based on erythema should be followed instead.

Treatment Interval (days)	Dose Adjustment
1 to 7	Hold dose or ↑ dose as per protocol
8 to 14	↓ dose by 25% of previous dose
15 to 21	↓ dose by 50% of previous dose
22 to 28	↓ dose by 75% of previous dose
> 28	Refer back to doctor, start over

Treatment of Specific Dermatoses

Psoriasis

Expected Outcome [B, IIa]

- Excimer laser and lamp phototherapies are about as efficacious as NBUVB phototherapy but with faster response time, resulting in lower cumulative UVB doses.
- Approximately 10 to 15 treatment sessions are required to achieve significant improvement (e.g. > 75% improvement).

Treatment Frequency and Duration after achieving Significant Improvement [C, IV]

- After achieving significant improvement, if the patient has started excimer light phototherapy three times per week during the clearing phase of treatment, depending on the response, the frequency of treatment sessions may be gradually reduced to two times per week for several weeks, followed by once per week for several weeks as maintenance therapy, and the treatment is then stopped finally.

Vitiligo

Expected Outcome [A, Ib]

- Many studies have shown similar clinical efficacy of both excimer laser and excimer lamp phototherapies for the treatment of vitiligo.
- Repigmentation can be noted as early as four weeks of treatment, after about 10 to 15 treatment sessions.About 80% of vitiligo patches show repigmentation after an average of 12 treatment sessions.
- Most efficacy studies involve treating patients on an average of 25 to 50 sessions; in others, more sessions are required. It is suggested that more treatment sessions may result in better repigmentation rates.

Treatment Frequency and Duration after achieving Significant Improvement [C, IV]

- After achieving significant improvement, if the patient has started excimer light phototherapy three times per week during the initial phase of treatment, depending on the response, the frequency of treatment sessions may be gradually reduced to two times per week for several weeks, followed by once per week for several weeks as maintenance therapy, and the treatment is then stopped finally.

Other Dermatoses [B, III]

- Atopic dermatitis (BSA < 5% involvement)
- Lichen simplex chronicus
- Hand dermatitis
- Patch-stage IA mycosis fungoides
- Alopecia areata
- Nodular prurigo
- Granuloma annulare

Further Reading

1. Cheng YP, Hsiu HY, Jee SH, *et al.* Excimer light phototherapy of segmental and non-segmental vitiligo: Experience in Taiwan. *Photodermatol Photoimmunol Photomed* 2012; 28: 6–11.
2. Feldman SR, Mellen BG, Housman TS, *et al.* Efficacy of the 308-nm excimer laser for treatment of psoriasis: Results of a multicenter study. *J Am Acad Dermatol* 2002; 46: 900–906.
3. Lapolla W, Yentzer BA, Bagel J, *et al.* A review of phototherapy protocols for psoriasis treatment. *J Am Acad Dermatol* 2011; 64: 936–949.
4. Le Duff F, Fontas E, Giacchero D, *et al.* 308-nm excimer lamp vs. 308-nm excimer laser for treating vitiligo: A randomized study. *Br J Dermatol* 2010; 163: 188–192.
5. Mudigonda T, Dabade TS, Feldman SR. A review of targeted ultraviolet B phototherapy for psoriasis. *J Am Acad Dermatol* 2012; 66: 664–672.
6. Mysore V. Targeted phototherapy. *Indian J Dermatol Venereol Leprol* 2009; 75: 119–125.
7. Park KK, Liao W, Murase JE. A review of monochromatic excimer light in vitiligo. *Br J Dermatol* 2012; 167: 468–478.
8. Passeron T, Ortonne JP. Use of the 308-nm excimer laser for psoriasis and vitiligo. *Clin Dermatol* 2006; 24: 33–42.
9. Taneja A, Trehan M, Taylor C. 308-nm excimer laser for the treatment of psoriasis: Induration-based dosimetry. *Arch Dermatol* 2003; 139: 759–764.
10. Zanolli MD, Feldman SR. *Phototherapy Treatment Protocols for Psoriasis and Other Phototherapy-Responsive Dermatoses*, 2nd ed. New York: Taylor & Francis Group; 2004.

Chapter

8

Photodynamic Therapy

Background

- Photodynamic therapy (PDT) involves the therapeutic use of a photochemical reaction generated from the interaction of a photosensitising agent, visible light and oxygen to selectively destroy targeted diseased tissue.
- In dermatology, the two most commonly used topical photosensitisers approved for PDT are 5-aminolaevulinic acid (ALA) and methyl aminolaevulinate (MAL). As MAL (Metvix®, Galderma) is used in our local practice currently, this chapter will therefore focus on MAL-PDT.
- After application of topical MAL cream to the skin lesion, there is preferential uptake and selective accumulation of MAL in the

more metabolically active cells such as the hyperproliferating malignant tumour cells.

- Being a prodrug, MAL is then metabolised in the haem biosynthetic pathway to the photoactive protoporphyrin IX (PpIX), which is subsequently activated by irradiating the skin lesion with light of a specific wavelength corresponding to one of its absorption peaks in the visible light spectrum (usually the red light). We use the Aktilite® CL128 (Photocure ASA) that produces narrowband red light with peak wavelength of 634 nm (Figure 7).
- The energy is then transferred to oxygen molecules to generate reactive oxygen species, which subsequently induce apoptosis and necrosis of the target cells. This is known as the photodynamic reaction.

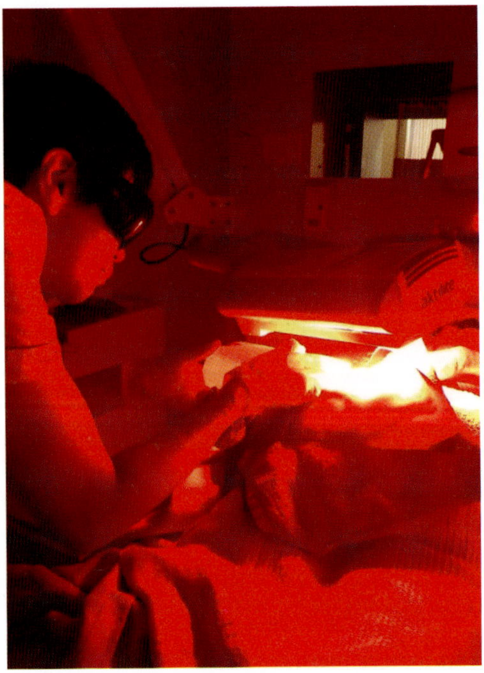

Figure 7. Irradiation with 634-nm red light (Aktilite® CL128) in photodynamic therapy.

Indications of PDT

Main

• Actinic keratosis	[A, Ia]
• Bowen disease	[A, Ia]
• Superficial basal cell carcinoma	[A, Ia]
• Nodular basal cell carcinoma	[A, Ia]

Others

• Acne vulgaris	[B, Ib]
• Viral warts	[B, Ib]
• Genital warts	[B, Ib]
• Cutaneous T-cell lymphoma	[B, III]
• Extramammary Paget disease	[C, III]

Contraindications to PDT

Absolute

- Porphyria
- Allergy to the active substance or any of the excipients in Metvix® cream such as arachis oil (peanut oil) and almond oil

Relative

- Pregnancy (Category C)
- Breastfeeding — should be discontinued for 48 hours after application of Metvix® cream

Adverse Effects of PDT

Acute

- Pain, including burning or stinging sensation
- Erythema
- Oedema
- Blistering
- Crusting

Chronic

- Post-inflammatory dyspigmentation
- Hair loss

Treatment Procedure

Stage 1: Lesion Preparation and MAL Application

1. Using a curette, gently remove surface scales and crusts adherent on the lesion. The surface of the lesion can be abraded further via dermasanding (dermabrasion). This allows better penetration of the MAL cream.
2. Debulking curettage is necessary for thicker nodular lesions, and this may require local anaesthesia using lignocaine (without adrenaline).
3. Apply topical MAL cream evenly on the prepared lesion using an applicator such as a spatula as a layer of 1 mm thickness. The cream should be applied beyond the edge of the lesion by 5-10 mm.
4. Cover the lesion with an occlusive dressing such as Tegaderm® (3M) followed by a light-protective dressing such as aluminium foil, which can be held in place with Micropore® (3M) tape.
5. Leave the occlusion in place for three hours, before moving on to Stage 2.

Stage 2: Irradiation with Red Light

1. Remove the dressing, wipe off the MAL cream and cleanse the area with 0.9% sodium chloride solution.
2. Check surface fluorescence using Wood's lamp in darkened room (fluorescence diagnosis). Record the presence and intensity of characteristic red fluorescence as follows:
   - 0 — no fluorescence
   - + — slight fluorescence
   - ++ — moderate fluorescence
   - +++ — strong fluorescence

3. Irradiate the lesion with Aktilite® CL128 red light lamp. The lamp is placed at a distance of 8 cm away from the target lesion. The total dose delivered is 37 J/cm^2. The irradiation time is approximately 8 minutes and 12 seconds, with the lamp irradiance of 75 mW/cm^2.

4. Ensure that the patient and nurse operating the lamp are wearing appropriate protective eyewear.

5. During the irradiation, measures that can be taken to reduce pain or discomfort include the following:

   - cool water spray
   - cooling fan
   - local anaesthesia, using lignocaine (without adrenaline)
   - regional anaesthesia (field block)
   - increase distance between the lamp and lesion

   For example, increasing the lamp-skin distance to 34 cm and setting the lamp dose at 74 J/cm^2 will deliver the same total dose of 37 J/cm^2, reduce the irradiance by half, but double the irradiation time.

6. After irradiation, repeat the fluorescence check to ensure that no fluorescence is detected. This is known as photobleaching. If residual fluorescence is detected, further extra irradiation of the red light at 18 J/cm^2 (equivalent to 50% of total original dose) is given. Repeat the fluorescence check to ensure photobleaching.

Post-PDT Care

1. Immediately after PDT, apply cold compress to relieve pain if necessary. An oral analgesic such as paracetamol may be taken as required.

2. Apply non-adherent dressing to protect the treated lesion from sun exposure.

3. Advise patient to protect the treated area from sun exposure for 48 hours after PDT to minimise any unwanted phototoxicity.

4. Apply white soft paraffin/petroleum jelly or octenidine gel regularly to minimise crusting and infection that may develop at the treated site.

5. Inform the patient that after PDT, burning or stinging sensation with some degree of pain, erythema and oedema may occur but these reactions are generally transient and of mild to moderate intensity. These reactions generally resolve within one to two weeks.

Follow-up

1. The MAL-PDT is repeated one week later. This constitutes one cycle of PDT.
2. Review the patient in three months, or earlier if necessary. MAL-PDT may be repeated at three months as the second cycle of PDT if the lesion has not completely cleared.

Summary of Treatment Evidence for the Main Indications

Skin Disorder	Efficacy	Recurrence	Cosmesis
Actinic keratosis	Clearance rate for two treatments of around 90%. Lower in acral sites. Comparative treatments ▪ Cryotherapy: 68–75% ▪ 5-fluorouracil: 70–75%	12-month recurrence rate of 16%. Comparative treatments ▪ Cryotherapy: 21% ▪ 5-fluorouracil: 18%	"Excellent" or "good" outcome for PDT (92–98%) vs. cryotherapy (51–75%).
Bowen disease	Clearance rate of around 90%. Comparative treatments ▪ Cryotherapy: 82% ▪ 5-fluorouracil: 83%	12-month recurrence rate of 15%. Comparative treatments ▪ Cryotherapy: 21% ▪ 5-fluorouracil: 18%	"Excellent" or "good" outcome for PDT (94%) vs. cryotherapy (66%) vs. 5-fluorouracil (76%).

(*Continued*)

Table (*Continued*)

Skin Disorder	**Efficacy**	**Recurrence**	**Cosmesis**
Superficial basal cell carcinoma	Clearance rate of 87–97%. Comparative treatments ▪ Cryotherapy: 82–95% ▪ Curettage and electrocautery: up to 97%	36-month recurrence rate of 6–22% (lower for small tumours < 1 cm). Comparative treatments ▪ Cryotherapy: 19% ▪ Surgery: 3–8% ▪ Curettage and electrocautery: 6–19%	"Excellent" or "good" outcome for PDT (87%) vs. cryotherapy (49%).
Nodular basal cell carcinoma	Clearance rate of 83–94%. Comparative treatment ▪ Surgery: 96–98%	60-month recurrence rate of 14–30%. Comparative treatment ▪ Surgery: 4%	"Excellent" or "good" outcome at five years for PDT (87%) vs. surgery (54%).

Further Reading

1. Alexiades-Armenakas M. Long-pulsed dye laser-mediated PDT combined with topical therapy for mild to severe comedonal, inflammatory or cystic acne. *J Drugs Dermatol* 2006; 5: 45–55.
2. Braathen LR, Szeimies RM, Basset-Seguin N, *et al.* Guidelines on the use of photodynamic therapy for nonmelanoma skin cancer:An international consensus. *J Am Acad Dermatol* 2007; 56: 125–143.
3. Coors EA, von den Driesch P. Topical photodynamic therapy for patients with therapy-resistant lesions of cutaneous T cell lymphoma. *J Am Acad Dermatol* 2004; 50: 363–367.
4. Dover JS, Bhatia AC, Stewart B, *et al.* Topical 5-aminolevulinic acid combined with intense pulsed light in the treatment of photoaging. *Arch Dermatol* 2005; 141: 1247–1252.

5. Fabbrocini G, Di Costanzo MP, Riccardo AM, *et al.* Photodynamic therapy with topical delta-aminolaevulinic acid for the treatment of plantar warts. *J Photochem Photobiol B* 2001; 61: 30–34.
6. Freeman M, Vinciullo C, Francis D, *et al.* A comparison of photodynamic therapy using topical methyl aminolevulinate with single cycle cryotherapy in patients with actinic keratosis: A prospective randomized study. *J Dermatolog Treat* 2003; 14: 99–106.
7. Kaufmann R, Spelman L, Weightman W, *et al.* Multicentre intraindividual randomized trial of topical methyl aminolaevulinate-PDT vs. cryotherapy for multiple actinic keratoses on the extremities. *Br J Dermatol* 2008; 158: 994–999.
8. Lehmann P. Methyl aminolevulinate-photodynamic therapy: A review of clinical trials in the treatment of actinic keratoses and nonmelanoma skin cancer. *Br J Dermatol* 2007; 156: 793–801.
9. Mori M, Campolmi P, Mavilia L, *et al.* Topical photodynamic therapy for primary cutaneous B-cell lymphoma: A pilot study. *J Am Acad Dermatol* 2006; 54: 524–526.
10. Morton CA, Horn M, Leman J, *et al.* A randomized, placebo-controlled European study comparing MAL-PDT with cryotherapy and 5-fluorouracil in subjects with Bowen's disease. *J Eur Acad Dermatol Venereol* 2004; 18: 415.
11. Morton CA, McKenna KE, Rhodes LE, *et al.* Guidelines for topical photodynamic therapy: Update. *Br J Dermatol* 2008; 159: 1245–1266.
12. Pariser DM, Lowe NJ, Stewart DM, *et al.* Photodynamic therapy with topical methyl aminolevulinate for actinic keratosis: Results of a prospective randomized multicenter trial. *J Am Acad Dermatol* 2003; 48: 227–232.
13. Schroeter CA, Pleunis J, van Nispen tot Pannerden C, *et al.* Photodynamic therapy: New treatments for therapy-resistant plantar warts. *Dermatol Surg* 2005; 31: 71–75.
14. Tarstedt M, Rosdahl I, Berne B, *et al.* A randomized multicenter study to compare two treatment regimens of topical methyl aminolevulinate-PDT in actinic keratosis of the face and scalp. *Acta Derm Venereol* 2005; 85: 424–428.
15. Wiegell SR, Wulf HC. Photodynamic therapy of acne vulgaris using methyl aminolevulinate: A blinded, randomized, controlled trial. *Br J Dermatol* 2006; 154: 969–976.

Chapter

9

Phototesting

Background

- Photodiagnostic testing is a method commonly used as an aid in the diagnosis, treatment and monitoring of a suspected photodermatosis.
- The test methods include phototesting, photopatch testing and photoprovocation testing, of which the most commonly utilised test procedure is phototesting.
- Phototesting is also used as an aid in determining the initial starting dose of the UVR during phototherapy or photochemotherapy.

Indications of Phototesting

Therapy

- The minimal erythema dose (MED) or minimal phototoxic dose (MPD) is determined to enable the selection of an appropriate starting dose to initiate NBUVB phototherapy or PUVA photochemotherapy.

Diagnosis

- In a case of suspected photosensitivity, the MED-UVA and MED-UVB are determined in order to classify the photosensitivity and hence to make a diagnosis.
- When there is an urticarial reaction, this is also documented.
- In solar urticaria, it is useful to determine the minimal urticaria dose (MUD) for UVA and UVB when there is a positive urticarial reaction, and document as such as MUD-UVA and MUD-UVB respectively.
- When there is a positive urticarial reaction to visible light (VIS), the MUD-VIS is then determined. If the light source is a slide projector, the duration or time taken for a positive reaction to occur is recorded instead of dose.

Monitoring

- It is useful to assess a patient's disease severity, and monitor the response to treatment and disease activity by serial determinations of MEDs and MUDs to UVA, UVB and VIS.

General Principles in Phototesting

Washout Period

- Application of topical corticosteroids and calcineurin inhibitors on the phototesting site should be stopped two weeks prior to phototesting.
- Systemic corticosteroids and immunosuppressants should be withheld four weeks prior to phototesting if possible.
- Oral antihistamines should be withheld one week prior to phototesting.

Anatomical Site

- For phototesting to determine the MED-UVA, MED-UVB, MED-NBUVB and MPD (in PUVA photochemotherapy), select an area of uninvolved skin from one of the following sites (in order of priority):

    1. Buttocks
    2. Lower back
    3. Abdomen (just above level of umbilicus, lateral to the midline)
    4. Upper back (axillary level, midway between posterior axillary line and spine)

- The buttock or lower back region is the preferred site for phototesting because of the relatively large area of skin available for phototesting and these sites are usually non-sun-exposed.

- For VIS phototesting, select an area of uninvolved skin that is non-sun-exposed, such as the inner arm, buttocks or lower back.

Irradiation Source

- For therapeutic phototesting, the UVR source used for testing is the specific irradiation source used for treatment. For instance, the NBUVB whole-body unit will be used for such phototesting to determine the MED-NBUVB when the same unit is used for phototherapy. Similarly, the UVA whole-body unit will be used for such phototesting to determine the MPD-UVA when the same unit is used for PUVA (oral or bath) photochemotherapy.

- For diagnostic phototesting, the flat-panel broadband UVA and broadband UVB canopy units can be used to irradiate the skin for determination of the MED-UVA and MED-UVB respectively (Figure 8).

- For VIS phototesting, the slide projector can be utilised as the VIS source to elicit any abnormal reaction, in particular an urticarial reaction (Figure 9).

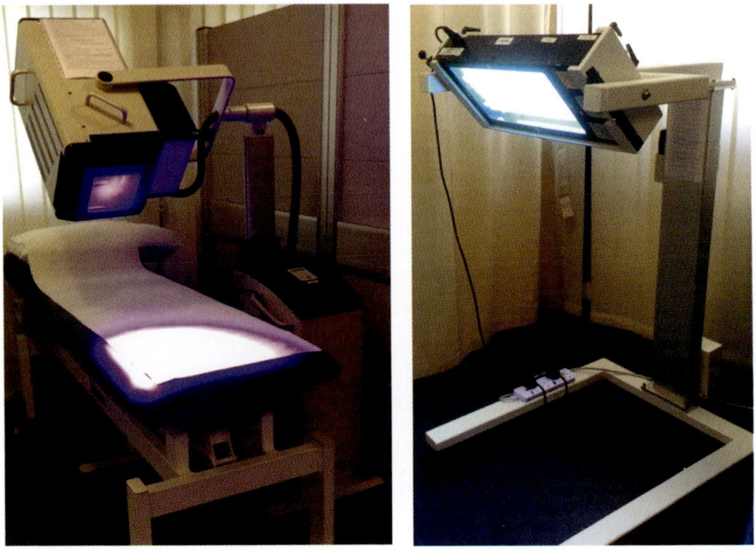

Figure 8. Broadband UVA (left) and UVB (right) canopy units used for irradiation during phototesting and photoprovocation testing.

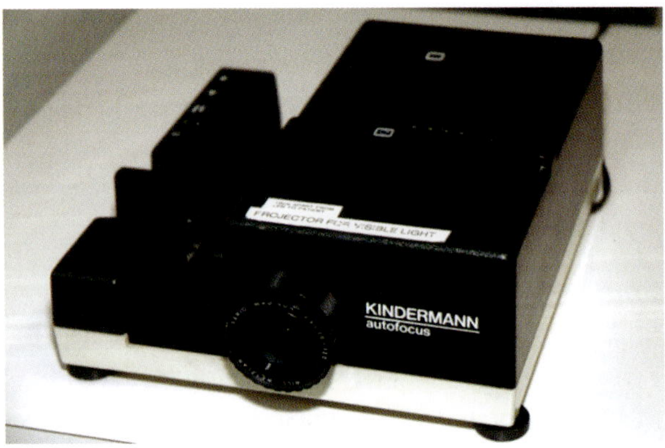

Figure 9. A slide projector can be used for VIS irradiation during phototesting.

- In the context of diagnostic phototesting, the broadband UVR sources and slide projector are referenced in this chapter to illustrate the phototesting procedure.

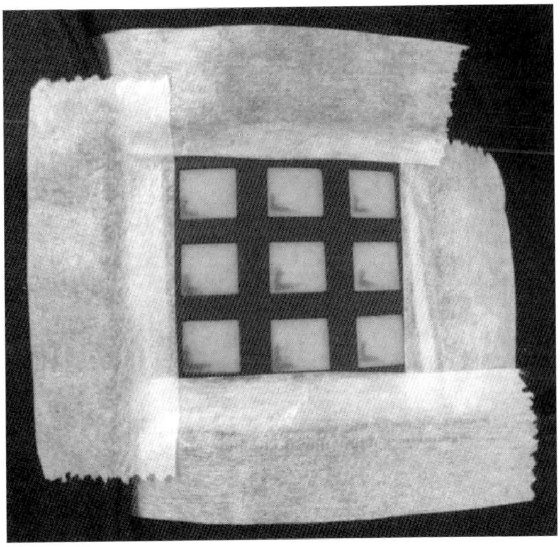

Figure 10. A UV-opaque template with nine apertures is attached to the phototesting site prior to irradiation.

Therapeutic Phototesting Procedure for NBUVB Phototherapy and PUVA Photochemotherapy [C, IV]

- Select an appropriate site that is non-sun-exposed, such as the buttocks or lower back.
- Other areas of the skin must be covered with layers of cloth made of UV-protective material.
- A template made of UV-opaque material, comprising nine square apertures, each measuring at least 1×1 cm size, is then attached to the pre-determined skin site (Figure 10).
- The location of each aperture is marked with a skin marker for easy identification.
- Ensure that the patient wears UV-protective goggles during UVR delivery.

- The dose for each aperture is dependent on the patient's skin phototype. Refer to Annexes A and B for details on MED testing and MPD testing dosimetry respectively.
- The dose delivery is performed by beginning with all of the apertures open for UVR testing and closing the individual apertures after a specific dose of UVR has been delivered using UV-opaque adhesive tape.
- At the end of the phototesting procedure, the template used in the phototesting is then removed and the areas rechecked to ensure that adequate marking of the skin has been done to identify the actual apertures tested.
- The patient is instructed not to wash or rub off the skin marks.
- It is essential that the patient is instructed not to expose the test area to any source of natural or artificial UVR till the return to the clinic for MED or MPD reading. The following table illustrates the various MED and MPD reading timings.

UVR	**MED/MPD Timing of Reading (hours)**
NBUVB	24
Oral PUVA	72
Bath PUVA	96

- When the patient returns to the clinic, the area of phototesting is identified by the markings at the different dose sites.
- The MED or MPD is defined as the dose of UVR that elicits an erythema that is just perceptible.
- Read the MED or MPD value and document the erythema response in each of the nine dose sites according to the following table.

Erythema Grading	Erythema Response
0	No erythema
±	Just perceptible erythema = 1 MED/MPD
+	Ill-defined erythema, pink
++	Well-defined erythema, flat
+++	Well-defined fiery-red erythema, palpable
++++	Well-defined fiery-red erythema with blistering

NBUVB Test Site Reactions

- If all test sites are positive and if the reaction to the lowest dose is very faint, the true MED will not be much below this and the lowest dose can be appropriately regarded as the MED.
- If all test sites are positive and if the reaction to the lowest dose is moderate to severe, MED testing may need to be repeated with a lower NBUVB dose series (see Annex A).
- If all test sites are negative, regard the highest test dose as the MED.

Oral PUVA Test Site Reactions

- If all test sites are positive and if the reaction to the lowest dose is very faint, the true MPD will not be much below this and the lowest dose can be appropriately regarded as the MPD.
- If all test sites are positive and if the reaction to the lowest dose is moderate to severe, MPD testing may need to be repeated after a lower oral dose of 8-MOP at 0.4 mg/kg and/or with a lower UVA dose series (see Annex B).
- If all test sites are negative, MPD testing should be repeated after a higher oral dose of 8-MOP at 0.6 mg/kg using the same UVA dose series.

Bath PUVA Test Site Reactions

- If all test sites are positive and if the reaction to the lowest dose is very faint, the true MPD will not be much below this and the lowest dose can be appropriately regarded as the MPD.
- If all test sites are positive and if the reaction to the lowest dose is moderate to severe, MPD testing may need to be repeated after a lower bathwater concentration of 8-MOP at 1.875 mg/L and/or with a lower UVA dose series (Annex B).
- If all test sites are negative, MPD testing should be repeated after a higher bathwater concentration of 8-MOP at 7.5 mg/L using the same UVA dose series.

Diagnostic Phototesting Procedure for UVA and UVB [C, IV]

- Select an appropriate site that is non-sun-exposed, such as the buttocks or lower back.
- Other areas of the skin must be covered with layers of cloth made of UV-protective material.
- A template made of UV-opaque material, comprising nine square apertures, each measuring at least 1×1 cm size, is then attached to the pre-determined skin site.
- The location of each aperture is marked with a skin marker for easy identification.
- The dose for each aperture is dependent on the patient's skin phototype. Please refer to Annex A for details on MED testing dosimetry.
- Position the UVA irradiation source above the pre-determined test site at a specific distance as recommended by the manufacturer.

- The source is then warmed up for a period that is recommended by the manufacturer.
- After the warm-up period, the phototesting procedure starts.
- The dose delivery is performed by beginning with all of the apertures open for UVR testing and closing the individual apertures after a specific dose of UVR has been delivered using UV-opaque adhesive tape.
- At the end of the phototesting procedure, the template used in the phototesting is then removed and the areas rechecked to ensure that adequate marking of the skin has been done to identify the actual apertures tested.
- At this stage when the procedure has been completed, a first immediate reading and a second reading at 30 minutes after the completion of the UVA irradiation are performed to assess for any urticarial reaction. When there is a positive urticarial reaction, this is then documented. Take note of the MUD. The MUD is defined as the dose of UVR that elicits a wheal that is just perceptible and palpable.
- Repeat the above phototesting procedure for UVB.
- When phototesting is completed for both UVA and UVB, the patient is instructed not to wash or rub off the skin marks.
- It is essential that the patient is instructed not to expose the test area to any source of natural or artificial UVR for the next 24 hours till the return to the clinic for MED reading.
- When the patient returns to the clinic, the area of the phototesting is identified by the markings at the different dose sites (Figure 11).
- The MED is defined as the dose of UVR that elicits an erythema that is just perceptible.

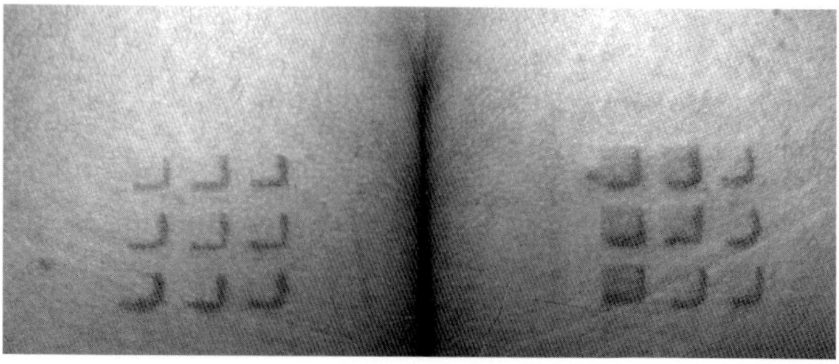

Figure 11. Phototesting performed on the buttocks, showing markings at the different dose sites representing incremental UVB (left) and UVA (right) doses.

- Read the MED value and document the erythema response in each of the nine dose sites according to the following table.

Erythema Grading	Erythema Response
0	No erythema
±	Just perceptible erythema = 1 MED
+	Ill-defined erythema, pink
++	Well-defined erythema, flat
+++	Well-defined fiery-red erythema, palpable
++++	Well-defined fiery-red erythema with blistering

UVA and UVB Test Site Reactions

- If all UVA and/or UVB test sites are positive and if the reaction to the lowest dose is very faint, the true MED will not be much below this and the lowest dose can be appropriately regarded as the MED.
- If all UVA and/or UVB test sites are positive and if the reaction to the lowest dose is moderate to severe, MED testing may need to be repeated with a lower UVA and/or UVB dose series (see Annex A).
- If all UVA and/or UVB test sites are negative, MED testing may be repeated with a higher UVA and/or UVB dose series to obtain the

actual MED values (see Annex A). This is particularly important in photoprovocation testing.

Diagnostic Phototesting Procedure for VIS [C, IV]

- Select an appropriate site that is non-sun-exposed, such as the inner arm, buttocks or lower back.
- Other areas of the skin must be covered with layers of cloth made of VIS-opaque material.
- A template made of VIS-opaque material, comprising one square aperture, measuring at least 2 × 2 cm size, is then attached to the pre-determined skin site.
- The location of the aperture is marked with a skin marker for easy identification.
- The slide projector is positioned 10 cm away from the test site, and the irradiation time is 20 minutes.
- A first immediate reading and a second reading at 30 minutes after the completion of the irradiation are performed to assess for any urticarial reaction. When there is a positive urticarial reaction, this is then documented (Figure 12).
- When the patient returns 24 hours later for the MED reading, any abnormal reaction at the VIS test site such as erythema or papular reaction is also documented.
- If there is a positive urticarial reaction at the VIS test site, determine the MUD-VIS by repeating the VIS phototesting procedure at the following shorter timings:
    - 1 minute
    - 2.5 minutes
    - 5 minutes
    - 10 minutes
    - 15 minutes

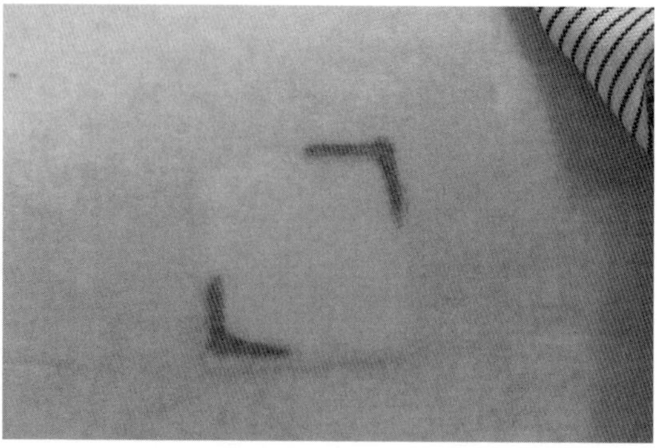

Figure 12. Phototest reading on the inner arm showing an urticarial response to VIS, consistent with solar urticaria.

- On the other hand, if there is a negative urticarial reaction at the VIS test site, and yet there is still a strong suspicion of solar urticaria, the VIS phototesting procedure can be repeated at the following longer timings:
    - 30 minutes
    - 40 minutes
    - 50 minutes
    - 60 minutes

Important Note on Solar Urticaria

- The sun emits UVR, VIS and also heat as infrared radiation (IRR). Thus, in the context of solar urticaria when there is a positive urticarial reaction seen in UVA, UVB and/or VIS phototesting, it is important to evaluate for heat urticaria as well, as heat urticaria may co-exist with solar urticaria.
- For further reading, the procedure of heat provocation testing can be found in:

  Magerl M, Borzova E, Giménez-Arnau A, *et al.* The definition and diagnostic testing of physical and cholinergic urticarias: EAACI/GA^{2}LEN/EDF/UNEV consensus panel recommendations. *Allergy* 2009; 64: 1715–1721.

Normal Ranges of MED-UVA and MED-UVB [C, IV]

- The following two tables illustrate the normal ranges of MED-UVA and MED-UVB according to skin phototype, adapted from *Fitzpatrick's Dermatology in General Medicine*.

Skin Phototype	Normal Range of MED-UVA (J/cm^2)
I	20–35
II	30–45
III	40–55
IV	50–80
V	70–100
VI	≈ 100

Skin Phototype	Normal Range of MED-UVB (mJ/cm^2)
I	15–30
II	25–40
III	30–50
IV	45–60
V	60–90
VI	90–150

Expected Phototesting Responses in Common Photodermatoses

- The following table summarises the expected phototesting responses in common photodermatoses.

Disorder	MED-UVA	MED-UVB	VIS	Action Spectrum
Polymorphic light eruption	Normal or ↓	Normal or ↓	Normal	UVA, UVB
Chronic actinic dermatitis	↓ or normal	↓ or normal	Normal or Erythema/ Papulation)	UVB, UVA (VIS)
Actinic prurigo	↓ or normal	↓ or normal	Normal	UVA, UVB
Hydroa vacciniforme	Normal or ↓	Normal or ↓	Normal	UVA, UVB
Solar urticaria	Normal ± urticaria	Normal ± urticaria	Normal ± urticaria	VIS, UVA, UVB
Drug-induced photosensitivity	↓ or low normal	Normal	Normal	UVA
Photocontact dermatitis	Normal	Normal	Normal	UVA

Further Reading

1. Farr PM, Dawe RS. Phototesting. In: Lim HW, Hönigsmann H, Hawk J, eds. *Photodermatology*. New York: Informa Healthcare USA; 2007.
2. Freedberg IM, Eisen AZ, Wolff K, *et al*. *Fitzpatrick's Dermatology in General Medicine*, 5th ed. New York: McGraw-Hill; 1999.
3. Macfarlane L, Bhoyrul B, Ibbotson SH. Practice when minimal phototoxic and minimal erythema doses are not determinable. *Photodermatol Photoimmunol Photomed* 2015; 31: 224–226.
4. Magerl M, Borzova E, Giménez-Arnau A, *et al*.The definition and diagnostic testing of physical and cholinergic urticarias: EAACI/GA^{2}LEN/EDF/UNEV consensus panel recommendations. *Allergy* 2009; 64: 1715–1721.
5. Rhodes LE, Friedmann PS.A comparison of the ultraviolet B-induced erythemal response of back and buttock skin. *Photodermatol Photoimmunol Photomed* 1992; 9: 48–51.
6. Yashar SS, Lim HW. Classification and evaluation of photodermatoses. *Dermatol Ther* 2003;16: 1–7.

Chapter

10

Photopatch Testing

Background

- Photopatch testing is the clinical investigation of choice in patients suspected of photoallergic contact dermatitis (PACD).
- It involves the application of suspected photoallergens on the skin followed by irradiation of UVA to induce photoallergic reactions (see Figure 13).

Indications of Photopatch Testing

- Suspected PACD
- Unexplained photosensitive eczematous eruption
- Chronic actinic dermatitis (CAD) or photoaggravated atopic eczema if there is unexplained worsening or no response to adequate therapy

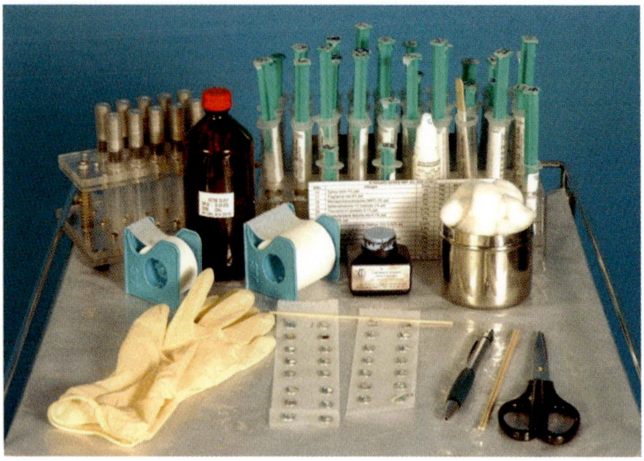

Figure 13. Photopatch testing allergens and equipment.

- Exposure dermatitis, or dermatitis predominant on exposed sites, when PACD needs to be excluded
- Skin intolerance to sunscreens
- Systemic drug photosensitivity, especially when systemic drug photochallenge is not feasible

Patient Preparation

Washout Period

- Application of topical corticosteroids and calcineurin inhibitors on the photopatch testing site should be stopped two weeks prior to photopatch testing.
- Systemic corticosteroids and immunosuppressants should be withheld four weeks prior to photopatch testing if possible.
- Oral antihistamines should be withheld one week prior to photopatch testing if photocontact urticaria is suspected.

Anatomical Site

- The preferred site for photopatch testing is located at the mid-upper back, at least 3 cm lateral to the vertebrae, avoiding the paravertebral groove.

- The test area should be free from active dermatitis for the preceding two weeks.

Irradiation Source

- The flat-panel canopy unit with fluorescent broadband UVA lamps can be used to irradiate the skin for photopatch testing as these lamps provide broad-spectrum output across the UVA region and the lamp irradiance is relatively uniform across a large irradiated site.

Photopatch Testing Series

- The various photopatch testing series differ among dermatology clinics and countries, depending on what the most commonly encountered photoallergens are in the respective clinics and countries.
- The suggested baseline and extended photopatch testing series provided in Annex C are adapted from the Sunscreen Series and the Scandinavian Photo Patch Series (Chemotechnique Diagnostics®).
- It is important to perform photopatch testing to the patient's own products as well.
- If exposure dermatitis is suspected, it is also essential to perform patch testing to standard series, any relevant series pertaining to the dermatitis, and the patient's own products.

Procedure for Photopatch Testing [B, IIb]

- On **Day 0**, allergens are first prepared in duplicates in Finn chambers on Scanpor tape, and these two identical sets of allergens are subsequently applied as parallel series on either side of the mid-upper back (Figure 14).
- On **Day 2**, both sets of allergens are removed from the back and discarded. The sites are then examined for reactions which are recorded using the International Contact Dermatitis Research Group (ICDRG) scoring system as shown in the following table.

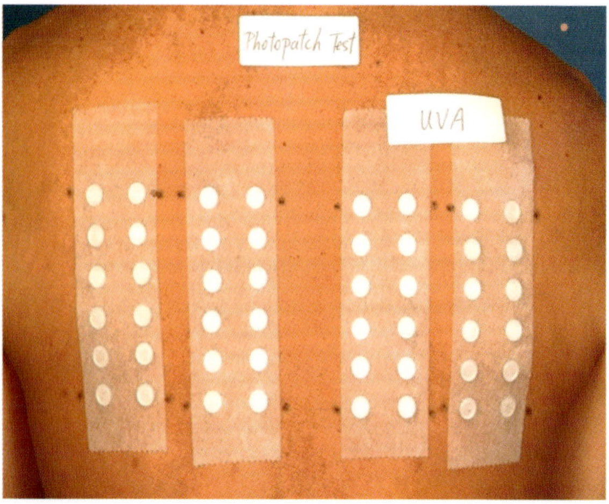

Figure 14. Allergens in Finn chambers patched on the upper back, duplicated on both sides (**Day 0**). UVA irradiation is then performed on the right side (**Day 2**).

Grading	Reaction
-	Negative reaction
?+	Doubtful reaction; faint erythema only
+	Weak positive reaction; erythema, infiltration, possibly papules
++	Strong positive reaction; erythema, infiltration, papules, vesicles
+++	Extreme positive reaction; intense erythema and infiltration, coalescing vesicles
IR	Irritant reactions of different types
NT	Not tested

- One set of sites (non-irradiated allergens) is shielded with UV-opaque material while the other duplicate set is irradiated with UVA (Figure 15).
- The generally accepted UVA dose is 5 or 10 J/cm^2. In our local context, due to the darker skin phototypes of our population, 10 J/cm^2 is used.
- Readings are performed immediately and 30 minutes after irradiation to assess for any solar urticaria that may be unexpected, and any suspected photocontact urticaria.

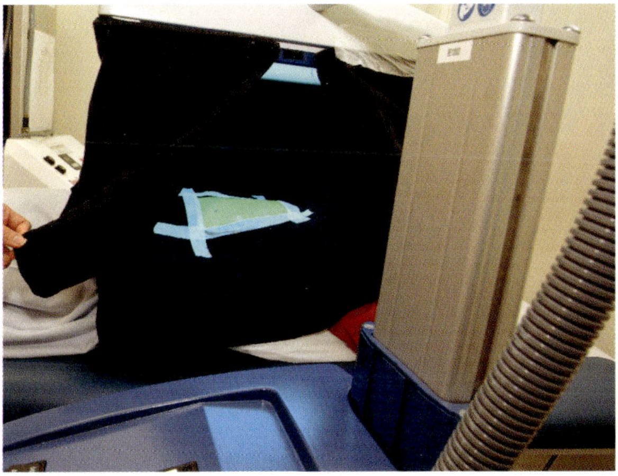

Figure 15. Irradiation on one side of the back with broadband UVA during photopatch testing.

- The patient is advised to wear dark-coloured, closely woven clothes and to avoid sun exposure.
- On **Day 4**, the sites are examined again for reactions which are then recorded.
- A further reading on **Day 6** or **7** is optional; it is more important when there is a need to differentiate a photoallergic reaction that exhibits a crescendo reaction pattern from a phototoxic reaction that exhibits a decrescendo reaction pattern, especially in the context of evaluating systemic drug photosensitivity.
- The following table illustrates a suggested schedule for photopatch testing.

Day 0	**Day 2**	**Day 4**	**Day 7 (optional)**
Monday	Wednesday	Friday	Monday
Application of allergens	Irradiate with 10 J/cm^2 of UVA; immediate reading	Reading	Reading; differentiate between photoallergy (crescendo reaction) and phototoxicity (decrescendo reaction)

Interpretation of Results

- The following table illustrates the various possible reactions that may occur during photopatch testing with their respective interpretations.

Non-irradiated site	Irradiated site	Interpretation
Negative	Negative	No allergy
Negative	Positive	Photoallergic contact dermatitis or Photoallergy (crescendo reaction pattern)
Positive	Positive Similar grade to non-irradiated site	Allergic contact dermatitis
Positive	Positive One or more grades stronger than non-irradiated site	Allergic contact dermatitis + Photoallergic contact dermatitis (or photoaugmentation of contact allergy)
Positive	Negative or Positive One or more grades weaker than non-irradiated site	Photoinhibition of contact allergy
Negative	Positive	Phototoxicity (decrescendo reaction pattern)

- When photoinhibition of contact allergy occurs, the photopatch testing is repeated for that particular allergen using 50% of the original UVA dose.

Documentation of Clinical Relevance

- The following table summarises the clinical relevance of the photopatch testing results.

Present relevance	The photopatch testing has unmasked an allergen that is causing the current dermatitis.
Past relevance	The photopatch testing has unmasked an allergen that has caused a dermatitis in the past, but the allergen is of no present relevance.
Past exposure	The photopatch testing has unmasked an allergen that the patient has encountered in the past, but at that time of exposure, the allergen did not produce a dermatitis.
Unknown relevance	No known exposure in the past; not sure if exposure is current or old.
Cross reaction	The positive photopatch testing is due to cross reaction with another allergen.

Complications

- Risk of sensitisation to allergens
- Flare of previous or existing dermatitis
- Irritant reactions from non-standard allergens or patient's own products
- Strongly positive UVA provocation at irradiated site of patients with CAD or UVA photosensitivity
- Dyspigmentation

Photopatch Testing in UVA-Sensitive Individuals [C, IV]

- It is advisable to determine the MED-UVA for a patient who is suspected of having UVA photosensitivity such as CAD, as a severe reaction may occur when the patient's skin is exposed to 5 or 10 J/cm^2. In this case, a false-positive photoexacerbated reaction is then interpreted as indicating photoallergy.
- The MED-UVA can be determined using the same UVA source as that to be used for photopatch testing.
- Photopatch testing can then be performed with UVA dose equivalent to 50% of the MED-UVA.
- Similarly, in a patient of unsuspected UVA photosensitivity when the photopatch testing has elicited a severe reaction at the UVA-irradiated test site, the patient's MED-UVA is then determined, followed by repeat photopatch testing with UVA dose equivalent to 50% of the MED-UVA.
- The following table illustrates a suggested schedule for photopatch testing combined with phototesting.

Day 0	**Day 1**	**Day 2**	**Day 4**	**Day 7 (optional)**
Monday	Tuesday	Wednesday	Friday	Monday
Application of allergens + Phototesting	MED reading	Irradiate with 50% of MED-UVA; immediate reading	Reading	Reading; differentiate between photoallergy (crescendo reaction) and phototoxicity (decrescendo reaction)

Further Reading

1. Bacthelor RJ, Wilkinson SM. Photopatch testing: A retrospective review using the 1 day and 2 day irradiation protocols. *Contact Dermatitis* 2006; 54: 75–78.
2. Bruynzeel DP, Ferguson J, Andersen K, *et al.* Photopatch testing: A consensus methodology for Europe. *J Eur Acad Dermatol Venereol* 2004; 18: 679–682.
3. Bryden AM, Moseley H, Ibbotson SH, *et al.* Photopatch testing of 1155 patients: Results of the U.K. multicenter photopatch study group. *Br J Dermatol* 2006; 155: 737–747.
4. Chuah SY, Leow YH, Goon AT, *et al.* Photopatch testing in Asians: A 5-year experience in Singapore. *Photodermatol Photoimmunol Photomed* 2013; 29: 116–120.
5. Duguid C, O'Sullivan D, Murphy GM. Determination of threshold UV-A elicitation dose in photopatch testing. *Contact Dermatitis* 1993; 29: 192–194.
6. European Multicentre Photopatch Test Study (EMCPPTS) Taskforce: A European multicentre photopatch test study. *Br J Dermatol* 2012; 166: 1002–1009.
7. Faurschou A, Wulf HC. Phototesting. In: Sterry W, Griffiths C, Korting HC, eds. *EDF Guidelines for Dermatology in Europe*. Berlin: ABW Wissenschaftsverlag; 2009.
8. Hasan T, Jansen CT. Photopatch test reactivity: Effect of photoallergen concentration and UVA dosaging. *Contact Dermatitis* 1996; 34: 383–386.
9. Ibbotson S. Photo-allergy and Photopatch Testing. In: Ferguson J, Dover JS, eds. *Photodermatology*. London: Manson Publishing; 2006.
10. Isaksson M, Bruze M. Photopatch testing. *Clin Dermatol* 1997; 15: 615–618.
11. Jansén CT, Wennersten G, Rystedt I, *et al.* The Scandinavian standard photopatch test procedure. *Contact Dermatitis* 1982; 8: 155–158.
12. Jindal N, Sharma NL, Mahajan VK, *et al.* Evaluation of photopatch test allergens for Indian patients of photodermatitis: Preliminary results. *Indian J Dermatol Venereol Leprol* 2011; 77: 148–155.
13. Photopatch testing: Methods and indications. British Photodermatology Group. *Br J Dermatol* 1997; 136: 371–376.
14. Pollock B, Wilkinson SM. Photopatch test method: Influence of type of irradiation and value of day-7 reading. *Contact Dermatitis* 2001; 44: 270–272.

15. Rietschel RL, Fowler JF. *Fischer's Contact Dermatitis*, 6th ed. Hamilton, Ontario: BC Decker; 2008.
16. Rosmarin D, Gottlieb AB, Asarch A, *et al*. Patch-testing while on systemic immunosuppressants. *Dermatitis* 2009; 20: 265–270.

Chapter

11

Photoprovocation Testing

Background

- Certain photodermatoses can be reproduced by repetitive exposure to ultraviolet radiation (UVR) and/or visible light (VIS).
- Photoprovocation testing aims to reproduce characteristic disease morphology on a localised area of skin after repeated exposure to a provoking wavelength or simulated sunlight.

Indications of Photoprovocation Testing

Diagnosis of Photodermatoses

- In suspected photodermatoses or photoaggravated dermatoses whereby the clinical picture is unclear and other tests have failed to provide diagnostic clues, such as in polymorphic light eruption (PMLE), chronic actinic dermatitis (CAD) and cutaneous lupus erythematosus (LE).

- Skin biopsy of the reproduced skin lesion can also be performed for confirmation of diagnosis of the photodermatosis.

Research

- Used in clinical trials to assess efficacy of potential photoprotective agents.

Patient Preparation

- Prior to photoprovocation testing, phototesting should be performed to document the MED-UVA and MED-UVB.
- The patient should be informed that a few consecutive visits are required during the photoprovocation testing as it involves daily UVR and/or VIS irradiations and reading of any positive reaction.
- Application of topical corticosteroids and calcineurin inhibitors on the photoprovocation testing site should be stopped two weeks prior to testing.
- Systemic corticosteroids and immunosuppressants should be withheld four weeks prior to photoprovocation testing if possible.

Procedure for Photoprovocation Testing [C, IV]

- The following photoprovocation testing procedure described is based on the same broadband UVA, broadband UVB and slide projector irradiation sources used in phototesting.
- After determining the MED-UVA and MED-UVB, calculate the UVA and UVB irradiation doses to be used during photoprovocation testing. The fixed-dose irradiation regimen is based on the following formula [B, IIa]:

UVA dose = 1.5 MED-UVA

UVB dose = 1.5 MED-UVB

- Photoprovocation testing for VIS is only performed for VIS-sensitive photodermatoses such as CAD. The time of VIS irradiation using the slide projector is set at 30 minutes.
- Select an appropriate site for UVA photoprovocation testing and attach a template made of UV-opaque material comprising one aperture measuring 5 × 8 cm in size to the pre-determined skin site. Repeat the same procedure for UVB and VIS photoprovocation testing.
- Other areas of the skin must be covered with layers of cloth made of UV-protective material.
- The location of each aperture is marked with a skin marker for easy identification.
- Photoprovocation irradiation commences on Day 1 (e.g. Monday) and continues daily for a maximum period of four days until Day 4 (e.g. Thursday), or until a positive reaction is seen.
- Readings are performed daily, 24 hours after each irradiation.
- If no positive reaction occurs during the four-day period of photoprovocation irradiation, further readings are performed at 24 hours after the last irradiation, i.e. Day 5 (e.g. Friday) and subsequently again at 96 hours, i.e. Day 8 (e.g. on the following Monday). If there is still no reaction seen, further readings are necessary if the photoprovocation testing is performed for the diagnosis of CAD (reading at one week) and cutaneous LE (readings at one, two and three weeks) after the last irradiation.
- Photoprovocation testing can be terminated earlier if clinical lesions appear before the completion of the 4-day irradiation. However, if the provoking wavelength is the subject of interest, photoprovocation testing to the wavelength that has not elicited a positive reaction can be continued up to a maximum period of four days, or until a positive reaction is seen.
- When there is a positive reaction, skin biopsy of the reproduced skin lesion can then be performed for confirmation of diagnosis of the photodermatosis.

- The following tables illustrate the photoprovocation testing protocols for various photodermatoses.

Photoprovocation Testing Protocol for PMLE

- Test site: area previously exposed, such as back and outer arms.

Day	UVA Dose (x MED)	UVB Dose (x MED)	Timing of Reading (hours)
1	1.5	1.5	—
2	1.5	1.5	24
3	1.5	1.5	24
4	1.5	1.5	24
5			24
8			96

Photoprovocation Testing Protocol for CAD

- Test site: uninvolved non-sun-exposed skin, such as buttocks and inner arms.

Day	UVA Dose (x MED)	UVB Dose (x MED)	Timing of Reading (hours)
1	1.5	1.5	—
2	1.5	1.5	24
3	1.5	1.5	24
4	1.5	1.5	24
5			24
8			96
11			One week after last irradiation

- VIS test site: set the time of irradiation using the slide projector at 30 minutes.

Photoprovocation Testing Protocol for Cutaneous LE

- Test site: back and upper forearms.

Day	UVA Dose (x MED)	UVB Dose (x MED)	Timing of Reading (hours)
1	1.5	1.5	—
2	1.5	1.5	24
3	1.5	1.5	24
4	1.5	1.5	24
5			24
8			96
11			One week after last irradiation
18			Two weeks after last irradiation
25			Three weeks after last irradiation

Systemic Drug Photochallenge [C, IV]

- Systemically administered drugs often reveal false-negative photopatch test results as the metabolites are likely to be the relevant photosensitisers instead of the topically applied test compounds themselves. Thus, systemic drug photochallenge may be a helpful test procedure in evaluating systemic drug photosensitivity.
- The route of administration of the drug during the systemic drug photochallenge is via the usual mode of administration, such as oral, subcutaneous, intramuscular or intravenous route.
- On <u>Day 1</u>, the drug is administered at a dose equivalent to twice the therapeutic dose. The same broadband UVA irradiation source used in photopatch testing is utilised in systemic drug photochallenge, delivering a constant dose of 10 J/cm^2 each time.
- The irradiation is performed on different test fields at the following timings:
    - Prior to drug administration
    - One hour after drug administration

- Two hours after drug administration
- Four hours after drug administration
- Eight hours after drug administration

- The procedure is modified from the photoprovocation test protocol and is described in the following table.
- Test site: back, five different test fields.

Day	Timing of Irradiation after Drug Administration (hours)	UVA Dose (J/cm²)	Timing of Reading (hours)
1	0	10	—
1	1	10	—
1	2	10	—
1	4	10	—
1	8	10	—
2			24
3			48
4			72
8			One week after last irradiation
15			Two weeks after last irradiation
22			Three weeks after last irradiation

Interpretation of Readings

- Photoprovocation testing is considered positive when typical lesions are elicited (Figure 16).
- The test is considered negative when there is no elicitation of typical lesions at the end of the reading period. However, a negative test result does not exclude the diagnosis of a photodermatosis.

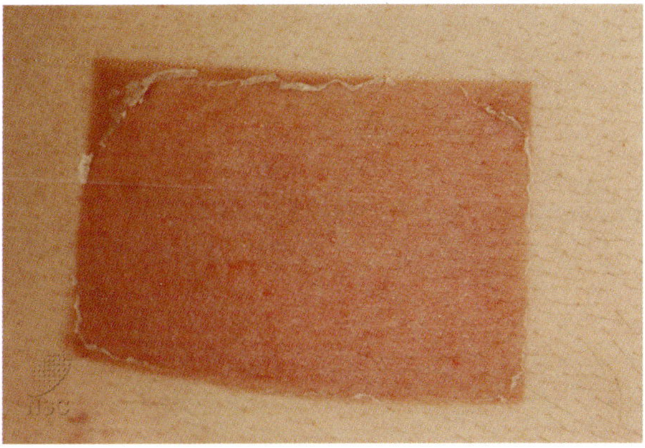

Figure 16. Photoprovocation testing with broadband UVB, showing tiny skin-coloured papules consistent with pinpoint papular polymorphic light eruption.

Complications

- Erythema
- Pain
- Pruritus
- Blistering
- Intense pigmentation and tanning that may last a few months, after repeated UVA and UVB irradiations
- Flare of underlying photodermatosis outside the irradiated sites

Further Reading

1. Akaraphanth R, Sindhavananda J, Gritiyarangsan P. Adult-onset actinic prurigo in Thailand. Photodermatol Photoimmunol Photomed 2007; 23: 234–237.
2. Chiam LY, Chong WS. Pinpoint papular polymorphous light eruption in Asian skin: A variant in darker skinned individuals. *Photodermatol Photoimmunol Photomed* 2009; 25: 71–74.

3. Krutman J, Hoenigsmann H, Elmets CA. *Dermatological Phototherapy and Photodiagnostic Methods*, 2nd ed. Berlin, Heidelberg: Springer-Verlag; 2009.
4. Kuhn A, Wozniacka A, Szepietowski JC, *et al.* Photoprovocation in cutaneous lupus erythematosus: A multicenter study evaluating a standardized protocol. *J Invest Dermatol* 2011; 131: 1622–1630.
5. Neumann RA, Pohl-Markl H, Knobler RM. Polymorphous light eruption: Experimental reproduction of skin lesions by whole-body UVA irradiation. *Photodermatol* 1987; 4: 252–256.
6. Sanders CJ, van Weelden H, Kazzaz GA, *et al.* Photosensitivity in patients with lupus erythematosus: A clinical and photobiological study of 100 patients using a prolonged phototest protocol. *Br J Dermatol* 2003; 149: 131–137.
7. Schmidt E, Tony HP, Bröcker EB, *et al.* Sun-induced life-threatening lupus nephritis. *Ann N Y Acad Sci* 2007; 1108: 35–40.
8. Schornagel IJ, Knol EF, van Weelden H, *et al.* Diagnostic phototesting in polymorphous light eruption: The optimal number of irradiations. *Br J Dermatol* 2005; 153: 1234–1236.
9. Stege H, Budde MA, Grether-Beck S, *et al.* Evaluation of the capacity of sunscreens to photoprotect lupus erythematosus patients by employing the photoprovocation test. *Photodermatol Photoimmunol Photomed* 2000; 16: 256–259.
10. van de Pas CB, Hawk JL, Young AR, *et al.* An optimal method for experimental provocation of polymorphic light eruption. *Arch Dermatol* 2004; 140: 286–292.

Annex

A

Minimal Erythema Dose Testing Dosimetry

Standard Dose Series for NBUVB

Modality	NBUVB		
Skin Phototype	**I/II**	**III/IV**	**V/VI**
Dose (mJ/cm²)	200	400	600
	400	600	800
	600	800	1000
	800	1000	1200
	1000	1200	1400
	1200	1400	1600
	1400	1600	1800
	1600	1800	2000
	1800	2000	2200

Lower Dose Series for NBUVB

Modality	NBUVB		
Skin Phototype	**I/II**	**III/IV**	**V/VI**
Dose (mJ/cm^2)	10	10	10
	25	25	25
	50	50	50
	100	100	100
		200	200
			400

Standard Dose Series for UVA

Modality	UVA		
Skin Phototype	**I/II**	**III/IV**	**V/VI**
Dose (J/cm^2)	2.5	5	10
	5	10	20
	10	20	30
	20	30	40
	30	40	50
	40	50	60
	50	60	80
	60	80	100
	80	100	120

Lower Dose Series for UVA

Modality	UVA		
Skin Phototype	**I/II**	**III/IV**	**V/VI**
Dose (J/cm^2)	1	1	1
		2.5	2.5
			5

Higher Dose Series for UVA

Modality	**UVA**		
Skin Phototype	**I/II**	**III/IV**	**V/VI**
Dose (J/cm^2)	100	120	140
	120	140	160
	140	160	180
	160	180	200
	180	200	220
	200	220	240
	220	240	260
	240	260	280
	260	280	300

Standard Dose Series for UVB

Modality	**UVB**		
Skin Phototype	**I/II**	**III/IV**	**V/VI**
Dose (mJ/cm^2)	2.5	5	10
	5	10	20
	10	20	30
	20	30	40
	30	40	50
	40	50	60
	50	60	80
	60	80	100
	80	100	120

Lower Dose Series for UVB

Modality	UVB		
Skin Phototype	**I/II**	**III/IV**	**V/VI**
Dose (mJ/cm^2)	1	1	1
		2.5	2.5
			5

Higher Dose Series for UVB

Modality	UVB		
Skin Phototype	**I/II**	**III/IV**	**V/VI**
Dose (mJ/cm^2)	100	120	140
	120	140	160
	140	160	180
	160	180	200
	180	200	220
	200	220	240
	220	240	260
	240	260	280
	260	280	300

Annex

B

Minimal Phototoxic Dose Testing Dosimetry

Standard Dose Series for PUVA

Modality	**Oral PUVA**			**Bath PUVA**		
Skin Phototype	**I/II**	**III/IV**	**V/VI**	**I/II**	**III/IV**	**V/VI**
Dose (J/cm^2)	0.5	1.0	1.5	0.25	0.5	1.0
	1.0	1.5	2.0	0.5	1.0	1.5
	1.5	2.0	2.5	1.0	1.5	2.0
	2.0	2.5	3.0	1.5	2.0	2.5
	2.5	3.0	3.5	2.0	2.5	3.0
	3.0	3.5	4.0	2.5	3.0	3.5
	3.5	4.0	4.5	3.0	3.5	4.0
	4.0	4.5	5.0	3.5	4.0	4.5
	4.5	5.0	5.5	4.0	4.5	5.0

Lower Dose Series for PUVA

Modality	Oral PUVA			Bath PUVA		
Skin Phototype	**I/II**	**III/IV**	**V/VI**	**I/II**	**III/IV**	**V/VI**
Dose (J/cm^2)	0.1	0.1	0.1	0.1	0.1	0.1
	0.25	0.25	0.25		0.25	0.25
		0.5	0.5			0.5
			1.0			

Annex

C

Photopatch Testing Series

Sunscreen Series (Baseline)

No.	Compound	Concentration % (w/w)	Vehicle
1	Butyl methoxydibenzoylmethane (Avobenzone, Parsol 1789)	10%	pet.
2	PABA (4-Aminobenzoic acid)	10%	pet.
3	Homosalate	5%	pet.
4	4-Methylbenzylidene camphor (Eusolex 6300, Mexoryl SD)	10%	pet.
5	Ethylhexyl dimethyl PABA (Eusolex 6007, Escalol 507)	10%	pet.

(Continued)

(Continued)

No.	Compound	Concentration % (w/w)	Vehicle
6	Benzophenone-3 (Oxybenzone)	10%	pet.
7	Ethylhexyl methoxycinnamate (Parsol MCX)	10%	pet.
8	Benzophenone-10 (Mexenone)	10%	pet.
9	Phenylbenzimidazole sulfonic acid (Eusolex 232)	10%	pet.
10	Benzophenone-4 (Sulisobenzone)	10%	pet.
11	Drometrizole trisiloxane (Mexoryl XL, Silatrizole)	10%	pet.
12	Octocrylene (Eusolex OCR)	10%	pet.
13	Ethylhexyl salicylate (Escalol 587)	5%	pet.
14	Ethylhexyl triazone (Uvinyl T 150)	10%	pet.
15	Isoamyl p-methoxycinnamate (Neo Heliopan E1000)	10%	pet.
16	Bis-ethylhexyloxyphenol methoxyphenol triazine (Tinosorb S)	10%	pet.
17	Methylene bis-benzotriazolyl tetramethylbutylphenol (Tinosorb M)	10%	pet.
18	2-(4-Diethylamino-2-hydroxy-benzoyl)-benzoic acid hexylester (Uvinul A+)	10%	pet.
19	Diethylhexyl butamido triazone (Uvasorb HEB)	10%	pet.
20	Disodium phenyl dibenzimidazole tetrasulfonate (Neo Heliopan AP)	10%	pet.

Photopatch Series (Extended)

No.	Compound	Concentration % (w/w)	Vehicle
1	Balsam of Peru	25%	pet.
2	Bithionol	1%	pet.
3	Chlorhexidine diacetate	0.5%	aq.
4	Chlorhexidine digluconate	0.5%	aq.
5	Chlorpromazine hydrochloride	0.1%	pet.
6	Diphenhydramine hydrochloride	1%	pet.
7	2,2'-Thiobis(4-chlorophenol)	1%	pet.
8	Fragrance mix I	8%	pet.
9	Hexachlorophene	1%	pet.
10	Promethazine hydrochloride	1%	pet.
11	Tetrachlorosalicylanilide (TCS)	0.1%	pet.
12	Triclosan	2%	pet.
13	Tribromosalicylanilide (TBS)	1%	pet.
14	Triclocarban (TCC)	1%	pet.

Key: pet. — petrolatum, aq. — water

Annex

D

Evidence Grading for Recommendations

Levels of Evidence

Ia Evidence obtained from meta-analysis of randomised controlled trials.

Ib Evidence obtained from at least one randomised controlled trial.

IIa Evidence obtained from at least one well-designed controlled study without randomisation.

IIb Evidence obtained from at least one other type of well-designed quasi-experimental study.

III Evidence obtained from well-designed non-experimental descriptive studies, such as comparative studies, correlation studies and case studies.

IV Evidence obtained from expert committee reports or opinions and/or clinical experiences of respected authorities.

Grade of Recommendation	Levels of Evidence	Criteria
A	Ia, Ib	At least one randomised controlled trial as part of the body of literature of overall good quality and consistency addressing the specific recommendation.
B	IIa, IIb, III	Availability of well-controlled clinical studies but no randomised clinical trials on the topic of recommendation.
C	IV	Evidence obtained from expert committed reports or opinions and/or clinical experiences of respected authorities. Indicates absence of directly applicable clinical studies of good quality.

Index